Thyme Essential Oil

The Farmacy Cabinet Series

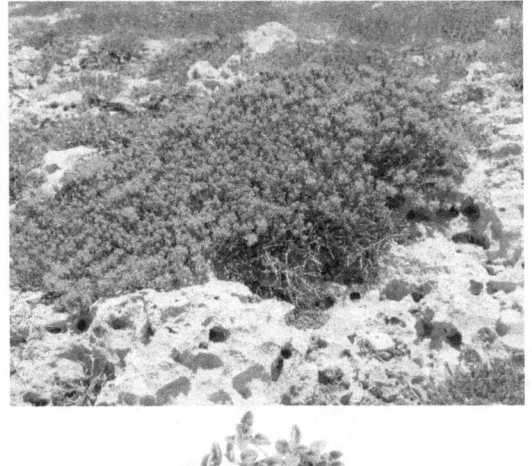

"…… 'Wellness' is found in Thyme"

Teach Your Children The Benefits of Essential Oils

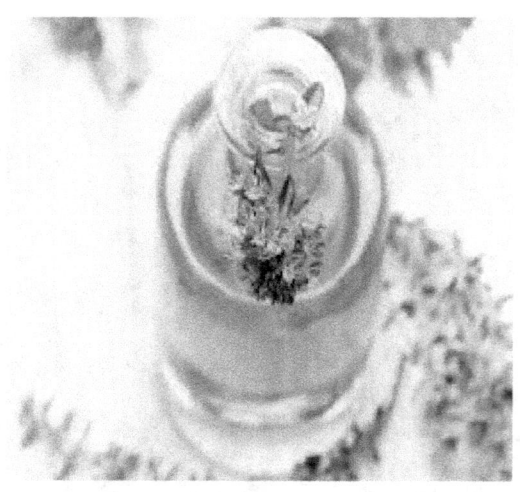

THYME
ESSENTIAL OIL
A FARMACY CABINET SERIES

First Edition
Karen L. Badea,
Certified Aromatherapist, CHt, RM

Copyright © 2015

Karen Badea

Karen L. Badea

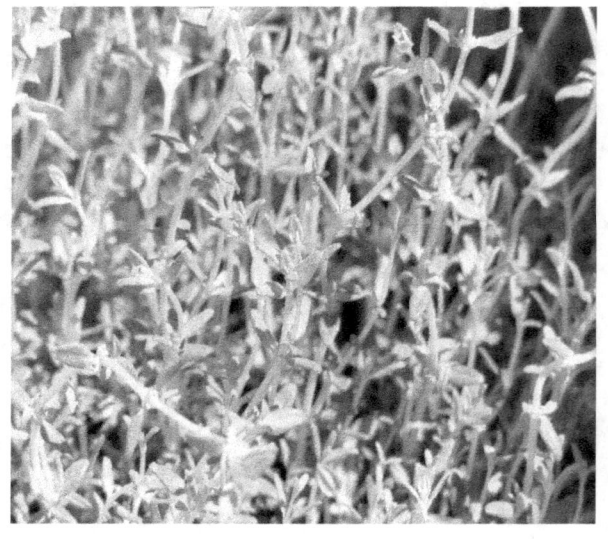

E-Published in the United States of America

ISBN: 978-1-5210-2662-5

eBook, 2015
Paperback, 2019

Table of Contents

Dedication

This book series is written for those interested in the healing power of essential oils. This is the first, of what I hope will become a long series of books on essential oils. Only through Chronic Lyme Disease has fate introduced me to these potent plants and the healing oils made from them. May your mind be open to research and to become your own health advocate. May you be awakened to the potent powers of what I call, 'God's Farmacy'…. I found a book out of 'happenstance' that sparked the interest level inside me enough to try essential oils as a form of treatment. My Lyme specialist had recommended a 'Lyme Essential Oil protocol' and I thought that he was just wanting to 'sell' me 'something'.

I bought the oils but never used them until I found a very special book and read it. It was a book written by an extremely knowledgeable professor and minister, Dr. David Stewart, entitled, 'Healing Oils of The Bible'. After reading this book and implementing the essential oils into my treatment protocols, my world improved beyond words. Yes, I decided to make the essential oils a healing avenue for my own chronic condition; just as my Lyme doctor had recommended a year earlier.

I am forever grateful for Mr. Stewart for writing and publishing such an informative biblical connection to the oils. Fore, those with a chronic condition, true natural healing knowledge means everything. We are tired of corporate 'money schemes' that result in draining our wallets and having no improvement, health wise. The oils have proven themselves tenfold in my healing journey. I hope you find essential oils to be of the same efficacy as I have….

Due to my positive medicinal experience with essential oils, I chose to become a Certified Aromatherapist and will continue my training to become a Registered

Aromatherapist. My dream was to become a medical doctor, but I was forced to change my degree and graduate earlier than planned, due to Lyme disease. Since then, I have come full circle in my Lyme healing journey. I have experimented and learned about a plethora of alternative health options. In fact, life dealt me an even better 'card'. As fate would have it, I diagnosed & tested myself for Lyme disease. I was positive and in 2013, I started the never-ending years of treatment for Lyme & coinfections. Lyme disease changed my life in so many ways. In fact, Lyme led me to learn the true form of medicine. It's called 'Nature'. Thus, I have found my 'niche' in life and it will be sharing the potent healing powers of alternative medicine, including herbs and essential oils to all that want to learn…So, in part, I dedicate this entire series to those fighting Lyme.

The first book in this series is specifically about Thyme and its healing components and properties. I converted a research paper, written for school, into my first Kindle book that will precede a series of additional books written about other healing essential oils. Yes, 'thyme' is one of my main preferred healing oils in my medicine cabinet and in my herb garden.

I feel thyme essential oil is vital to anyone's healing tool cabinet. Thyme has a special spot in my personal life, of which I will explain later... Blessings to all that fight chronic health conditions, and may they find their 'wellness in thyme'…

This was the last known photo that I have of my 'Paw' & I together…. My aunt had bought me a bathing suit and they wanted to take a photo of me. I wouldn't take the picture unless my 'Paw' was in it…. I remember that day like it was yesterday, yet it was nearly 50 years ago…….

Keep in mind, this is my first published work on Amazon Kindle. I saw a need for written educational material on individual oils. Many of the EO books that I have seen, cover a multitude of oils. I want to offer a specialized series of books that focus each book on an individual oil.

I pray that I only improve in my writing and research skills…. I wish to dedicate my first book to my maternal grandfather, Charles Wesley Pike, whom loved me more than life itself. He passed when I was only 6 years old, but his love lives on in my heart forever…".

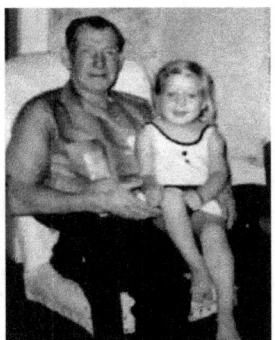

Love ya, Paw" ….

~Karen B

Disclaimer

I am not a professional licensed health practitioner, lawyer, nor 'undertaker' and in no way is anything in this publication meant to prevent, diagnose, treat, nor cure any health condition.

This information is for educational purposes only. One must see a licensed health practitioner for all health inquires. In addition, all persons, corporations, suppliers, educational venues, etc.... mentioned within this report, are not affiliated with me, personally, in any way, nor I, with them. I am merely mentioning some for educational purposes. One must decide independently what sources they will use as authorities in their own professional practice or for personal wellness objectives. I do not take responsibility for any information used in this book, nor will the entities mentioned, herein, take responsibility for the information in this book. Nothing herein is meant to be interpreted as advice. You are responsible for your own health and educational choices. Therefore, it is paramount that you research wisely and speak with your health provider on all health issues.

Please be advised that the material herein is not guaranteed to be correct, nor complete. You must do your own research and speak with your physician before making healthcare decisions.

"We must turn to nature itself, to the observations of the body in health and in disease to learn the truth."
~Hippocrates

Foreword

Here's to your exploration of THYME ESSENTIAL OIL...

However, before one can understand the oils, they must understand the herb itself, its growth process, its many components, and its many uses around the globe. In order to understand an essential oil; one must dive deep into the constituents of the plant that provides the oil.

You may have heard the old saying, "Thyme in the garden is precious thyme, indeed."……Well, I made my own 'saying' to prove the point that it is very important to learn the differences of thyme, even when the name stays the same. Hence, "Thyme in your garden may be quite different than thyme in mine." By this statement, I am trying to show you that not all thyme is alike. Not even if its species is the same… I want to show you that different varieties or Chemotypes, of an herb like thyme, can result in a plethora of various components being found in a plant that may have the same name, yet be made with varying percentages of healing components…. Hence, your essential oil needs to be thoroughly tested to know what the main components are in the plants that comprise the essential oils that you use or sell to clients. One cannot know the Chemotype by just saying the 'name' alone. We must know the conditions that produces each Chemotype. I hope to discuss a broad spectrum of data about the herb, thyme, in general.

I feel one must know a subject thoroughly to become an expert in that subject. Therefore, that means that not only will I speak of thyme essential oil in this book, but also of the herb that is used to make the oil, including a few other uses of thyme, besides being used to make essential oil. We will review the importance of knowing organic components individually and recognizing their medicinal values within the essential oil. I will be including a short summary of the main components and their basic medicinal values. Fore, the dominant percentage quantities of those components are what makes one variety of thyme better than other varieties for specific illness issues. As a professional Aromatherapist that works with clinical cases, knowing the fine details of each essential oil is very important. Hence, it is in the fine details, that we will have success in our profession. In fact, our professional success is measured by the healing experiences of our clients using the essential oils that we prepare and recommend.

Over the last year, I've found many essential oils to be useful in my own personal healing journey with chronic Lyme. I've especially found thyme essential oil, to be very potent and full of great therapeutic value. Keep in mind, essential oils are up to 70% stronger than the herb itself. [1] Thyme essential oil is a tremendous addition to my medicinal protocols. Finding my way back to wellness from chronic Lyme and its nasty, deadly co-infections has been a journey, indeed. It has been a journey that I would not wish on my worst enemy. It is a journey that many fight indefinitely. Thyme helps many chronic issues.

Moreover, as I evolve on my pathway to wellness, I realize the healing values of many other essential oils, in addition to thyme essential oil. They include frankincense, myrrh, oregano, cinnamon, and a special blend sold by Young Living, called 'Thieves'.

The 'Thieves' special blend is often sold with a similar themed name by competitive essential oil companies. For instance, Plant Therapy calls a similar blend, 'Germ Fighter'. I use this often. The original name idea came from France, of which the recipe is on display at the Louvre. This is a blend made famous by thieves surviving the plague during the 1400's. In addition to those oils that I have already mentioned above, black pepper, grapefruit seed oil, cedarwood, melaleuca, lavender, sandalwood, clove, and black seed oil, etc.... are also potent healing oils. (Keep in mind that BLACK SEED OIL is not an essential oil because it has a fatty lipid. It is an oil used in the Bible and I use it as my carrier oil for all the other essential oils used in massage. I use black seed oil daily, both externally & internally.)

Each oil has its own unique healing constituents that make it medicinally valuable. Research is proving that essential oils can, indeed, lower antibiotic use. Not to mention, pathogens do not mutate into an immune strain so easily using nature's essential oils versus replicated chemical antibiotic options.

Although it takes a multitude of essential oil components to treat a complex chronic disease, Thyme's amazing therapeutic attributes are to be commended above many of today's traditional mainstream therapies (One can source

PubMed, and other peer reviewed databases, to see the many studies that prove Thyme's medicinal efficacy). Yes, this small, tender, feminine-like plant makes some very potent essential oil. Thyme is respected by many physicians, as one of God's herbal medicinal miracles. Thyme spreads as a perfect, lush, green, ground cover and makes any garden look as if it were a 'prize winning' oasis.

Thyme's tiny green leaves and plethora of sprigs jut out across the floor of my herb beds. It is beautiful to behold anytime one stops to gaze at the multitude of medicinal plants growing in my personal backyard.... I have many wildcraft plants also in my garden;

transplanted from the Appalachian Mountain ranges in WV, VA, KY, and NC.

As for the size of the plant, itself, it depends upon the species. Some thyme tends to bush out to about a 9-10" maximum; while other varieties grow low and meander like a tightly knit green carpet. In the US, thyme grows best in zones 5-9 and loves full sun wherever it grows. [2] It usually has a very pleasant aroma, but there are some varieties that have no aroma (T. pseudolanuginosus, also known as, 'Woolly thyme'). [3]

I enjoy gathering my thyme and bringing it inside to process in my kitchen. By freezing it, I can preserve both its aromatic and healing components. However, I dry much of my thyme for use in my own homemade soaps, teas, soups, & tinctures. This fantastic little herb is used in a variety of ways from culinary to medicinal purposes. After studying the different percentages of organic components found in various thyme species, I have come to realize that one herb alone, like thyme, can have MANY specialized healing benefits depending on, the genus, where it is geographically grown, conditions of its environmental growth cycle, and when it is harvested.

Moreover, one needs to realize that when they are shopping for any essential oil, they need to know that even though the species of plant may be the same name, the constituents in that essential oil, will vary according to the multiple variables mentioned above. Hence, this is where we get the term, 'Chemotype', meaning an herb that can produce varying dominance of organic components in various percentages. This ability to produce varying degrees of components is all because these plants can adapt easily to their environmental conditions.

Thus, in this book, I will cover some rather interesting informational tidbits about the herb, thyme. I will explain thyme's harvesting process, the internal organic components found in various Chemotypes, and the use of various Chemotypes for medicinal purposes. I've even thrown in a few interesting little recipes at the end of this book. They are both culinary and medicinal recipes using fresh thyme in culinary dishes and, of course, using thyme essential oil in various recipes.

I've also added a small bonus for anyone wanting to know more about becoming a Certified or Registered Aromatherapist. I sincerely hope that I will have 'wet your whistle' about essential oils and aromatherapy, after reading this book. At least, enough to pursue an in-depth research of the healing capabilities of the oils.

Getting back to my original quote of, "Thyme in your garden may be very different from thyme in mine", which is my way of bringing CHEMOTYPES found specifically in the herb, Thymus vulgaris, to your attention. It is of vital importance for all Aromatherapist to request proper data spectrometry analysis (GC/MS) reports from all oil suppliers. Fore, as professional Aromatherapist, we must know the exact percentages of components found in every essential oil that we use or sell to clients. This is like a pharmacist, whom must know the ingredients, side effects and safety precautions of each drug they dispense to customers.

Here we go, please don't let this information overwhelm you if you are not the 'sciency' type. ("Sciency?" ...hmmm, that isn't a word, but you get the point.) Just continue reading the info slowly and digest it as you read. Note that all this 'CHEMOTYPE' info is important when learning how to use Thyme and other EO for their greatest benefits. So, keep in mind that there are some varieties of plants that have the same name but are considered to have a multitude of different 'Chemotypes' (CT). These plants with the same genus, yet different 'Chemotype' vary according to what component is found to be the most dominant in that particular plant (Even though the genus is the same, there are the variables of component dominance to take into consideration before recommending an oil for a particular medicinal use). For example, Thymus vulgaris CT thymol is used differently than Thymus vulgaris CT linalool. The thymol CT is used as a strong anti-microbial, whereas, CT linalool is often used in bathing, with children, and to calm mild anxiety. The individual component variances dictate what their best medicinal use will be. So, I repeat again, Thyme has several Chemotypes.

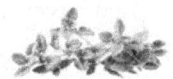

"The person who takes medicine must recover twice, once from the disease and once from the medicine."
~ William Osler, M.D.

My Personal Introduction to Thyme

Before I get started writing about one of the most precious plants in my herb garden, as well as, one of the top 5 healing oils in my medicine cabinet, I want to let you in on my herbal history and 'why' I chose thyme oil as my research for this; my first book ever published.

I was in my 30's before I had ever heard of the herb, 'thyme'. Now that is embarrassing to admit, but I was raised on a tobacco farm, in the middle of rural Kentucky. My parents always had a large garden, but herbs were not part of our lives. In fact, the word, 'herb' was not even in my vocabulary during my childhood years. (That would have been considered, "talking fancy", according to my mother. After all, I was a child of not just the south, but of the rural knob lands of Kentucky......tobacco farmers. Our main staples were fried potatoes, pinto beans, and cornbread. We didn't know too much about domestic garden 'herbs. My grandmother used wild weeds from the Appalachian mountain ranges and the fields on the farm in Kentucky.)

She did use sage in Thanksgiving dressing, and we used dill seeds in pickles when we canned, but herbs were never introduced to me outside of those two occasions and I didn't even realize they would have been called an 'herb'. Then, one day in my early 30's, while touring this cute little cottage for sale, I saw the word, 'Thyme' painted on a wooden sign. The sign hung above the garden gate at the side of the house. It was the highlight of the cottage's side entrance to a beautiful, well-kept garden, surrounded by a pristine white picket fence.

Immediately upon returning home after touring the cottage, my curiosity got the best of me, so I started researching to see what the word, 'Thyme' meant and what it was all about. (I seriously had no clue).

In my research, I found a photo of thyme and fell in love with the plant. I planted my first herb that following Spring, and yes, it was 'Thyme'. Regardless, of my new awareness of this one herb, 'herbal knowledge' was not widespread in my area of Kentucky, not in my 'tobacco farm circle' anyway. It wasn't until I went to work on the cruise ships, that I learned about several culinary herbs.

Over the years that I was working in the restaurant department of the cruise industry, I made friends with several Executive chefs and Sous chefs in the galleys. The cruise industry will indeed awaken one's culinary awareness and herbal vocabulary very quick.

A few years later, I married a European chef in Romania and was introduced to the various herbs, teas, and tinctures used for medicinal purposes in Eastern Europe.

After our marriage, my kitchen has since been full of fresh and dried herbs. My husband is the one whom started my true education in herbs. He was full of knowledge of herbs, tinctures, home remedies, etc…. I then started growing a variety of herbal plants in my own backyard. Today, 10 years later, we always have fresh, frozen, or dried herbs accessible at our home. In fact, I have a drying rack on wheels that my husband built, and it is full of thyme, sage, & mint, as I write this paragraph.

As I mentioned previously, I was diagnosed in 2013 with Lyme & several deadly co-infections. I was shocked when my Lyme Literate MD encouraged me to use essential oils to help heal myself. At first, I felt he was trying to sell me something' and I still was holding on to the thought that the oils were 'inferior' to my expensive 'big pharma' antibiotics. At the time, I was taking over $5000 monthly of various antibiotics and immune building supplements. Regardless, I must admit, my Lyme doctor did make me curious as to wanting to find out the reasons 'why' these oils were such powerful healing agents.

By this time, I was fully aware of the culinary embellishments that herbs brought to our food but was still not versed on the healing molecules in essential oils. I kept thinking, "there must be something to these oils or a doctor would not risk their professional reputation." One day while scrolling online to buy a Kindle book about essential oils, I came across a very interesting title. This book was written by Dr. David Stewart and entitled, 'Healing Oils of The Bible'. The title alone sparked my curiosity even more. I went on to order and read a second book, also written by Dr. David Stewart, 'The Chemistry of Essential Oils Made Simple'. [4] Wow, I was hooked on the oils.

I had always been interested in medicine and had plans of attending medical school before I was diagnosed with Lyme. Although, at the time, I didn't realize I had Lyme, yet, I knew something was seriously wrong.

Hence, I was forced to change degrees and graduate early due to my illness. I thought my dreams of becoming a 'healer' were forever gone. Little did I know that my true healing journey was just beginning at that point.

I've always heard that God works in mysterious ways, and he certainly had a plan for me. I feel royally blessed to have been introduced to the world's healthiest healing substances (aka essential oils). My new journey has introduced me to the medicinal benefits of essential oils, just as God promised in the Bible:

However, as I mentioned above, I first thought my Lyme specialist was 'trying to make money on selling me essential oils'. Yet, after a few more months of taking such expensive antibiotics and anti-helminth protocols, I

was still not feeling any great improvements. Not even after weeks of antibiotics via a PICC line. So, I realized that if I were to ever heal, I had to find 'something more'. After reading Dr. Stewart's books and better understanding the 'science' of the oils, I was eager to give them a chance.

Ahh, at last, I found relief and improvement after only a week of ingesting and massaging specific essential oils that were known to help with my health dilemma. I give complete credit to God's gift of healing essential oils. Fore, they literally gave me back a defined amount of quality to my daily life… Although, I still seek complete healing, the oils remain one of my main daily protocols.

I'm still in the treatment phase, but I can drive again and go places occasionally. I have noticed that with months of essential oil treatment, it's as if the Lyme bacteria has harbored or sandwiched into my fascia area between the dermal layers of my skin and the muscle tissues. I've read where this area of the body has less oxygen and that Lyme spirochetes thrive in an oxygen free environment. Regardless, of my Lyme journey, essential oils have been responsible for my improvement from constant seizures and being bedridden 24/7. I stayed in tremors, often, until I introduced essential oils into my daily treatments.

Moreover, it was easy to see that the EO's were much more potent, in my case, than my previous protocols. Therefore, I made the decision that I wanted to learn as much as possible about these healing oils and their medicinal benefits. I was hooked on the efficacy and I decided to find the best educational venue to educate myself on the healing powers hidden inside all essential oils.

Therefore, after carefully researching to find the best, most affordable, school to attend, I chose Aromahead Institute to complete my Aromatherapist certification. I was very pleased with the curriculum and the online learning experience. Furthermore, when it came time to write my final research paper, I thought it appropriate to write it on the essential oil that is derived from that first herb I was ever introduced too, 20 years prior...THYME.

Yes, I remember well that wooden sign, hanging above a garden gate in Perryville, KY…It simply had the word, 'Thyme' painted in green. My, how my life has unfolded over the years since then... I've literally sailed around the world and back, many times, since first being introduced to the word, THYME…

Surprisingly, here I am today, converting a school research paper into my first self-published book and remembering the first time I met 'thyme'. I can only hope that the 'The Farmacy Cabinet Series' will help to educate those like myself that want to learn the medicinal traits of plants.

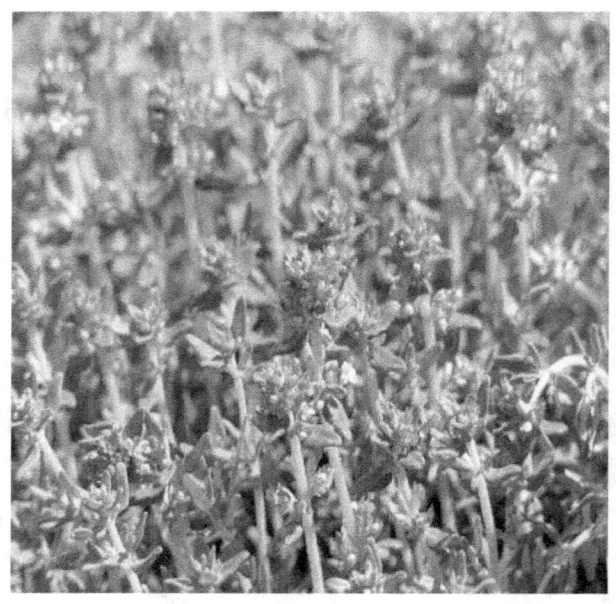

"And by the river upon its bank, on this side and on that side, shall grow all trees for food, whose leaf shall not fade, neither shall its fruit be consumed: it shall bring forth new fruit according to its months, because the waters flowed out of the sanctuary: and its fruit shall be for food, and its leaf for medicine."
~ Ezekiel 47:12

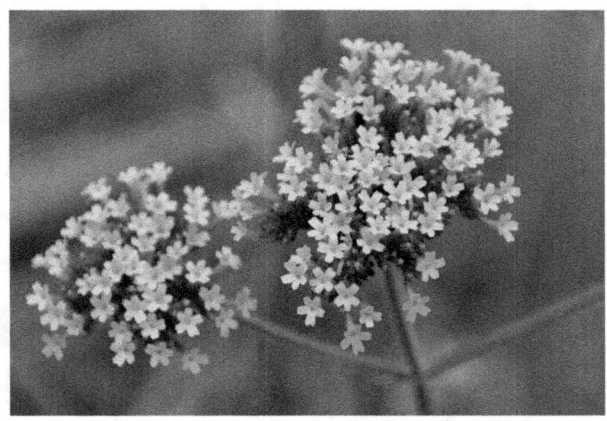

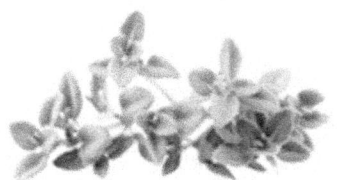

"In the midst of the street of it, and on either side of the river, [was there] the tree of life, which bare twelve [manner of] fruits, [and] yielded her fruit every month: and the leaves of the tree [were] for the healing of the nations."
~ Revelation 22:2 KJV

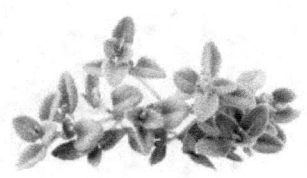

"We each have the innate ability to heal ourselves.
To empower ourselves with natural solutions,
instead of succumbing to life-altering chemicals.
There's a time and place for pharmaceuticals, but it
shouldn't be the first answer, nor the only form of
treatment."
~Dana Arcuri

Origins of Thyme

In my research, I have found the meaning of Thymus vulgaris, a common species of thyme, to originate from two very different words. Some say its origin is related to the word 'thymon', which is of Greek origin, meaning 'to fumigate', while 'vulgaris' originates from the Latin word meaning, 'common'.

Thyme belongs to the Lamiaceae family. Mint belongs to this same family. [5] Thyme is an aromatic low growing herb that looks like a shrub or can be a flat growing matt of tender tangled vines with tiny green leaves...Thyme does produce a flower, as well. Please note that most thyme essential oils found in the United States will be produced from the common thyme species, Thymus vulgaris.

In addition, Thymus vulgaris has several Chemotypes, of which I will discuss later. Even though the name is the same, the Chemotypes are determined by not only the elevation, time of harvest, but also by the environmental conditions and soil that the plant is grown in.

Don't be mistaken by thinking that only the 'common' form of thyme, Thymus vulgaris, is the ONLY variety of thyme that has healing components. Other Thymus

species, found throughout the planet, have fantastic healing constituents in them also and are used daily for specific medicinal purposes. Component percentages found in other varieties of thyme are different from the common variety of, 'Thymus vulgaris', yet just as healing, if not more, for certain health conditions.

As for the origins of thyme essential oil, the herb originated in Spain, but can be found in the Middle East, Europe, North America, and North Africa. 1200 meters above sea level seems to be the magic prime growth level. The countries that excel in thyme essential oil commercial production are Spain, Morocco, India, Switzerland, and of course, France. France, being the origin of the 'creme de la crème' of thyme essential oils. However, hardier varieties are making commercial growth possible for farmers in the northern latitudes of the planet, including North America. [6]

There is so much to share about the properties of thyme essential oil. It's complexity of varied components are a book in themselves. I hope that this book will give a basic idea of just how essential oils are such a great benefit in the medicinal arena. Indeed, I hope that your understanding of thyme essential oil and how important it is to healing protocols is much clearer after reading the info herein.

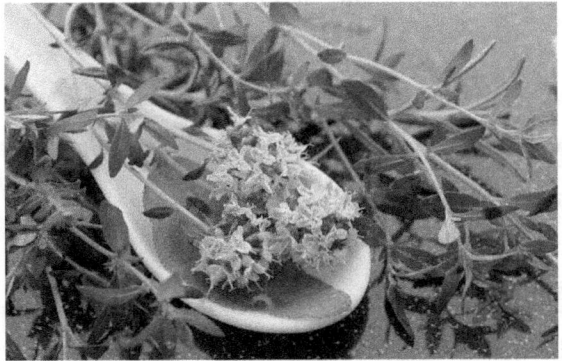

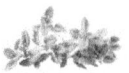

"Leave your drugs in the chemist's pot if you can heal the patient with food."
~Hippocrates

History of Thyme Use

To start out with a bit of historical info on this miraculous herb, thyme was mentioned as a respiratory aid in the famous, 'Hippocratic Corpus'. This ancient work, according to Wikipedia.org, was thought to possibly be from a collection in the Library of Cos, or even written in Alexandria, during the third century before Christ. Although, it is not a sure thing that Hippocrates, himself, even had anything to do with this precious ancient medical scroll. [7]

Regardless, thyme holds a special spot on this medicinal scroll, named after Hippocrates. Even before Hippocrates, the Egyptian culture was known to use thyme as an embalming agent, as well as, a culinary flavoring. [8] Whereas, the Ancient Greeks used thyme as a spiritual element in their holy temples by burning incense made from thyme. In fact, thyme has possibly been used since the beginning of time'. The Sumerians were known to have used the herb thyme over 3500 years ago. [9]

One of the oldest historical references of thyme was found in, 'The Kahun Gynaecological Papyrus', the oldest known medicinal reference in the world, dating back to 1800 BCE. This papyrus was mainly written for female medicinal purposes but mentioned various herbs in the last portion of the ancient artifact. Thyme was on the list of herbs mentioned in the papyrus and was specifically used for pain relief during that time period. [10]

Only through my research did I find information on thyme being used in Baby Jesus's manger, mixed within the hay. [11] It was supposedly used for aromatic reasons. Also, it has been used historically to preserve meat, as well as, to flavor liqueurs, cheeses, etc.… It was even once used on bandages to help in the healing process of wounds.

Furthermore, I found thyme also mentioned in Hildegard' Medicine, a German medicinal written work by Hildegard of Bingen (1089-1179), whom was a Benedictine herbalist. [12]   As you can see, thyme has been a medicinal force for thousands of years.

Yes, thyme has been part of human history and is still used widely in our world today. Thyme is a very potent healing substance. Today, however, thyme's medicinal benefits have been proven by scientific peer reviewed experiments. The healing components inside any essential oil are no longer

thought to be 'witchery'. The efficacy has been proven and science has learned the individual scientific healing powers of the individual organic components found within plant essential oils. Today, around the world, essential oils are found in a plethora of home medicine cabinets. Make sure you add THYME ESSENTIAL OIL to your FARMACY CABINET.

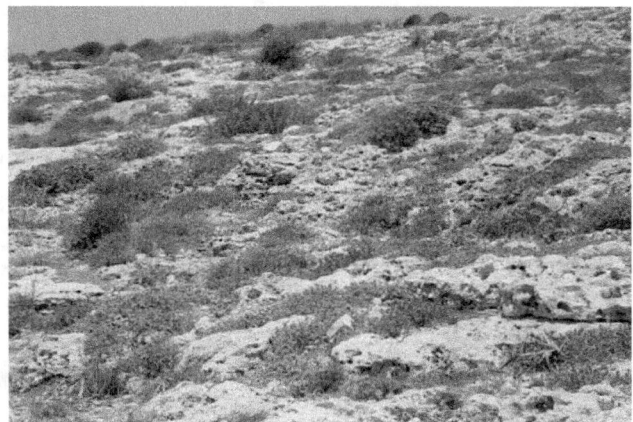

NOTE: Women wore thyme in their hair throughout history to catch the eye of a suitable beau. The single girls loved wearing thyme because it was a way of showing femininity.

"The Herbs ought to be distilled when they are in their greatest vigor, and so ought the Flowers also."
~Nicholas Culpeper

Storage & Quality Importance

Preservation of this precious herb is vital to its healing efficacy. There are special measures taken to keep this herb fresh or to keep the oils from oxidizing. In order to keep this herb at its freshest, the shelf life can be extended when in a 0 Celsius temperature range. [13] To process and retain its freshness, coating the thyme herb with canola oil as soon as possible after harvesting, will inhibit browning of the herb. The harvested herb can also be frozen and kept for up to one year.

Packaging thyme is best in glass or metal to prolong the aroma. Keep note that the quality of the healing components in the herb, will diminish over time, so it is vital to keep them sealed well and in a dark cool place. Thyme oil made via steam distillation also purifies the oil or sterilizes it, to be used for medicinal purposes. Hence, thyme, indeed, holds a special place throughout the ages in the medicinal and spiritual aspects of people's lives… Therefore, proper storage and processing is paramount to insure medical efficacy.

Dark glass bottles, either brown glass or blue, are best for storing your thyme essential oil. Most distributors will mail your product in one of these colored bottles with a dropper top. Make sure to tighten the top after each use. Again, keep your bottles in a cool, dark place for longer potency. Make sure labels are legible on all bottles.

One very important bit of information is to make sure that your essential oil bottles all stand up and are not laying ontheir sides. If allowed to lay on their side, the oils often seepout of the bottle and touch the rubber dropper at the top of the bottle. If this should happen, the oils will decompose the rubber dropper top. This destroys the oils and the dropper.

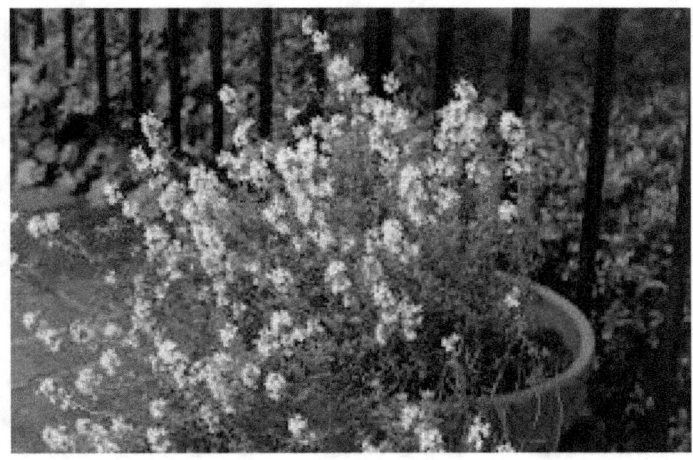

"Do not follow where the path may lead. Go, instead, where there is no path and leave a trail."
~Ralph Waldo Emerson

Resources & General Info on Thyme

I've found many sources of information on thyme while doing the research for this project. One of the most influential sources I found, is the book entitled, 'Thyme: Genus of Thymus', by Elisabeth Stahl-Biskup and Francisco Saez. [14] This book is an exceptional research tool for the professional Aromatherapist, and it describes approximately 350 varieties of thyme found on Earth. There are more than just the 350 mentioned in this book.

However, the book has a good grasp of the main ones available to the western world, as well as, those on the Eastern side of the globe. (There are some varieties that may not be as readily available, possibly due to political or economic reasons, like the one I will mention later from Iran.)

The species that Ms. Biskup and Mr. Saez, have chosen to be included in their book, are mainly species that originated in Europe and North Africa. They mention the fact that commercial distributors are mainly found within the European Union. Yet, North America and

Canada are currently expanding their thyme production by researching winter savvy plants.

The book, 'Thyme: Genus of Thymus', is a bit expensive on Amazon; priced at approximately $157 for a paperback version the last time I checked. Especially, since it is noted as the most comprehensive book written on the entire scope of thyme production...

So, instead of purchasing this book, I called my local library and requested an interlibrary loan to use as a source for this report. Indeed, I plan on purchasing this book eventually for my own private library and to also have as a tool for future students that I plan on teaching essential oil wellness classes too. In fact, I hope to find similar quality resources for each of the healing oils that I plan on writing about. I tell you how I borrowed via interlibrary services to give you an idea to do the same if you need special info on any oil research. It can save you tons of money.

(In addition to the source above, I have found such priceless information by searching PubMed and Medline for peer reviewed articles involving the use of thyme essential oil used for medicinal purposes. These too, are 'must' sources for the professional Aromatherapist. There is a plethora of studies done involving various varieties of thyme essential oil. These studies have proven that thyme essential oil, in general, has a high efficacy rate in treating pain relief, the immune system, digestive, respiratory, and even nervous system issues.)

Thyme essential oil is normally steam distilled from the dried or fresh flowers, leaves, and sometimes the stem of the plant. The flowers have nectar and are used by bees to make honey. Thyme's healing efficacy has always been well known throughout history, but 'big pharma' has stifled the information from the educational and medical systems of today. Recently, however, the increased interest in natural health options has caused the essential oil industry to 'skyrocket' in sales and educational interest. The entire industry is exploding right now, with many farmers & wineries entering the essential oil distillation business, as well as, Naturopaths and Aromatherapist that prescribe or recommend essential oils for medicinal purposes to patients or clients.

There are huge global multi-level marketing companies selling essential oils and this 'word of mouth' type sales model is bringing the essential oil information to the most remote rural areas of the country. Moreover, many rural cultures, as well as, the Amish and Mennonites, have been using these oils for centuries; long before the big 'MLM's' even existed.

Regardless, of the new buzz, about essential oils in many health-conscious homes, the use of essential oils and other alternative protocols has long been forgotten in many families, as the elders of the family pass. Convenience and 'educational conditioning' to 'big pharma' have rendered the younger generations captive to 'the corporate system'.

For, the truth remains, that for each generation that passes, our ancestors have taken their profound knowledge of natural healing with them to their grave. The corporations that produce chemical synthetic medications profit as each generation passes. Fore, the younger generations know very little about natural protocols.

However, recently, via social media and 'word of mouth' (MLM sales model), the essential oil industry is, indeed, booming. Society is tired of the chemical medications that seem to only treat symptoms, cause serious, sometimes deadly, side effects, and are so expensive that many deplete their entire life savings, in their quest to regain health.

Many of these 'big pharma' medications cause worse side effects (even death in many cases) than the condition they hope to treat.

You can verify this by reading the drug pamphlets included in your medications. Therefore, one of the very reasons that essential oils are becoming the medicinal 'choice' of many before going to the doctor for antibiotics. The essential oils do not have these serious side effects that the pharmaceuticals present. Thyme essential oil is one of the top healing oils and every medicine cabinet needs to have a supply of various Chemotypes of this miracle oil.

The average citizen is often oblivious to where they can purchase the essential oils and they need to have a Certified/Registered Aromatherapist to guide them on the medicinal use of such essential oils and also to furnish the oil blends that their condition may benefit from… After all, blending essential oils involves a well-trained Aromatherapist, who is educated in the constituents of each oil. The components in EO's often work in synergistic formats. The medicinal efficacy can often be doubled, if the oils are blended correctly.

Quality is paramount when using an Essential oil of any kind. Asking for the GC/MS data sheets from your supplier is vital to giving your customer the purest oil possible. Many distribution companies or 'middlemen' are boosting their profit line by blending carrier oils or synthetic components with the pure oils before shipping to you. This is the 'dirty' part of the EO industry. It's mainly found on the distributor level and not the distillation level.

Dr. Robert Pappas, PhD, known as a global authority on EO chemistry, has been known to randomly check top brand oils and find synthetics in what was labeled and sold as a pure oil. He has worked as a third-party consultant for 2 of the top MLM EO companies. Moreover, I have completed Dr. Pappas's EO chemistry lectures on YouTube where he is teaching the first and only Essential Oil Chemistry class at Indiana University. He has a very useful free website that is called Essential Oil University. http://essentialoil.university/. [15]

I highly recommend learning all that you can from Dr. Robert Pappas. He offers the same paid course via Essential Oil University website.

Should you decide to venture into growing your own garden spot full of Thyme, or even a container of Thyme, remember that this plant grows best with a rocky terrain, both at root level and also on the top of the soil. Make sure your soil has no peat. Many gardeners or essential oil producers know that germination is quite difficult with the Thyme seed, therefore germinating them inside where the temperature is 70 degrees consistently gives your success rate a boost.

Make sure that you have plenty of rock and drainage once you plant them permanently. Who knows, you may even have such success with this plant, that you might consider planting commercially with winter hardy thyme plants. One can sell the young plants themselves locally to nurseries, sell the herb fresh for culinary purposes, dry the herb for culinary, process and package for the supplement industry, choose to dry for later essential oil distillation to larger distillers, or use the plants fresh from the fields for essential oil distillation yourself.

Thyme will retain its essence and culinary strength better in dried form than many other plants. The demand for such a popular medicinal and culinary oil definitely exists and has proven to be extremely beneficial, economically to our global economy.

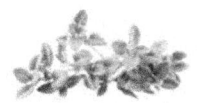

Karen L. Badea

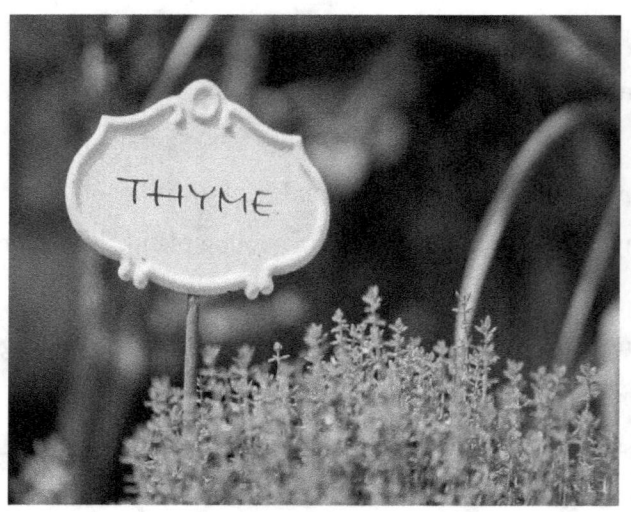

"Let thy food be thy medicine and thy medicine be thy food."
~Hippocrates (460-377 B.C.)

Chemotypes of Thyme

I promised to mention the Chemotypes of the common form of Thymus vulgaris. There are several. It is important to note that the most important aspect of component dominance depends on the elevation that the plant grows. Many variables determine the final Chemotype dominance in a plant.

For example, terpenes synthesis happens in the chloroplast of the plant. Therefore, light has much to do with the content of terpenes in the end product, as well as, moisture, time of harvest, sea level, etc.... [16] I have mentioned the main Chemotypes below, along with some 'notes' on that particular Chemotype. THYME is one of the most valuable medicinal plants WIDELY used in Pharmacology.

When purchasing essential oils, the label often, but not always lists the CHEMOTYPE. I buy many of my oils from Plant Therapy and they do list the chemotype. Some of the major MLM companies may not list chemotypes.

Just do your research before you purchase the oils to make sure you are buying the best product. The 'best' is not always the most expensive.

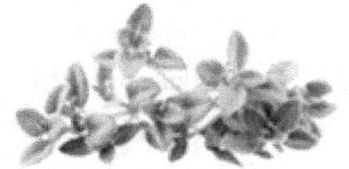

Thymus vulgaris CT thymol (2-isopropyl-5-methylphenol)

(Red Thyme) Can cause skin irritation for some. Skin test the person first. This CT is bountiful during Fall harvest. Usually grows at sea level. Great antibacterial properties. Very strong hot oil. Ranks 1st in frequency levels of components in Thymus. Thymol can be made synthetically. It is one of 'THE' most beneficial substances in the pharmaceutical industry. There is a long list of health 'conditions' treated with thymol. It's found in soaps, shampoos, toothpastes, deodorants, and even in mouthwashes. It is known to address inflammation and lower cytokines. Thymol was also used by the Egyptians in mummification.

Thymus vulgaris CT carvacrol

If harvested in the Fall, there can be as much as an 80% carvacrol content. Ranks 2nd in frequency levels for Thymus behind thymol. Carvacrol is a substance that has been used throughout history as a folk medicine remedy. It is found not only in Thyme, but also in Oregano, Black Cumin, Savory, and Pepperwort. Black Seed Oil (aka Cumin) is even mentioned in the Bible. Note that Carvacrol is often made synthetically, as well. Make sure you buy ORGANIC THERAPEUTIC THYME OIL so that you avoid the synthetic fillers.

Thymus vulgaris CT linalool

(Garden Thyme) This is the mildest of Thyme oils and availability is low. It has terpene alcohol linalool dominance. 3rd ranking in frequency for Thymus components. Often collected by hand, which contributes to higher expense, as well as, having a low yield, which also contributes to a higher cost. Today, this oil is mainly cultivated at 1200ft above sea level in the country of France. This oil is a pale-yellow color and is considered much milder than some of the other Chemotypes of Thymus vulgaris. Linalool is much milder than White Thyme and is the better option to use if treating a child.

Thymus vulgaris CT p-cymene

Unique in it must be harvested in the Spring while it is budding, BUT if not harvested in the SPRING, then it must be considered a thymol CT. Grows just above sea level, above the CT thymol. Ranks 4th in component frequencies for Thymus.

Thymus vulgaris CT alpha terpineol

This CT has a pepper like aroma and must be part of Spring production. 5th ranking frequency level for components found in Thymus.

Thymus vulgaris CT borneol - (Moroccan origin)

Ranks 6th in frequency levels for Thymus. Has a drug interaction with blood coagulant medications. It is a very unique oil due to its borneol content. It is highly effective in chronic infectious disease situations. The borneol is known to be able to "downregulate pathologically elevated levels of gamma globulins as they occur in many chronic conditions." http://aromatherapycouncil.org/nt,

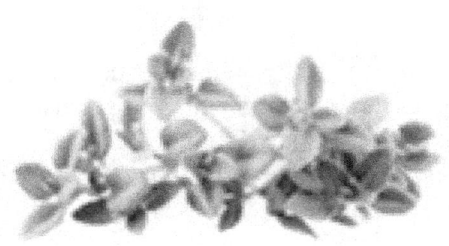

Thymus vulgaris CT 1,8 cineole

Ranks 7th in levels of frequency for components found in Thymus. (Great for insect repellents and has more carvacrol than Eucalyptus globules).

Thymus vulgaris CT geraniol

(Lemon Thyme) It is grown at high altitudes. Can possibly react with medications that use the CYP2B6 enzyme to metabolize. Fall harvest. Rarest of Chemotypes found in Southern France. [17]

Thymus vulgaris CT phenol

This CT is found in the Northern areas of the planet (Red Thyme) Can cause skin irritation for some. Skin test first. Fall harvest. Usually grows at sea level. Great antibacterial properties. Very strong hot oil.

Thymus vulgaris CT thujanol

(Sweet Thyme) This CT is only wildcrafted. Immune stimulant. Found mainly in the wild. However, this CHEMOTYPE of thyme is so high in demand that many producers are producing from cloned plants now. This oil was proven by a British University to kill Chlamydia.. Contains terpene alcohol thujanol. This Chemotype is considered a middle note scent. It blends especially well with Roman chamomile, lavender, bergamot, rosemary, geranium, and the citrus essential oil family. [19]

As I mentioned, the 'CT' or Chemotype refers to the component found to be dominant in that particular plant. Obviously, there are many Chemotypes (CT) for Thymusvulgaris, as I have listed above. Please don't confuse these

CT as being the only components in that oil. There are many components found in each CT, with a variety of percentages in each. The CT simply refers to 'the' particular component that is dominant in the plant material used for making that specific essential oil.

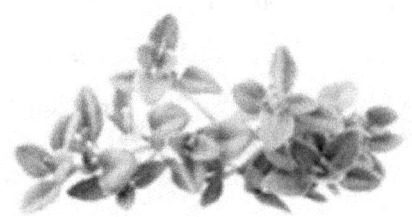

Again, the dominance factor is determined by environmental conditions during the growing process, the elevation, the soil content, moisture availability, the amount of direct sunlight, season it was harvested, and the variety of plant. There are plants with no Chemotype, which means that that particular plant doesn't have the ability to adapt to its environment like the plants that can alter their composition according to the threat they may be experiencing during their development process. Each constituent has been studied in a plethora of studies for its individual best medicinal benefit. Each Chemotype is harvested at different times in the growth process to assure the desired dominant component is at par level for what it is meant to treat.

Some components are even recognizable by simply smelling the plant leaf itself. Ever wonder 'why' so many Chemotypes? I have asked this same question many times, myself. It has been suggested that it could be a variation according to what chemicals the plant deemed necessary for defense purposes from parasites, insects, etc... in the location they are growing. Another possible reason is thought to be that the different components found in the plant itself, may have different energy requirements to produce the various percentages of dominance. Thus, resulting in applicable Chemotypes. [20]

The most common forms of thyme found in the western world are Thymus vulgaris, Thymus zygis, and Thymus serpyllum (Wild Thyme or Serpolet). [21]

The pleasant aroma of Thymus vulgaris is possible due to the plants many strong hair-like glands that reside on the leaves of the plant itself. Volatile oils in these glands will disseminate into the air when the glands are crushed by a hand, knife, or press, etc... This is why the room is full of aromatic smells when thyme is being chopped in our kitchens. Thyme continues throughout the summer exuding its aromatic scent in the gardens around our homes. There are a couple different types of glands in the leaves that contain the essential oils. One type has essential oils in the upper glandular cells and the other contains oils in the base cells of the leaf.

These oils are high in monoterpenes, a prime healing component in many of the Mediterranean essential oils. Thymus vulgaris grown in Egypt often has a high thymol & carvacrol concentration during the beginning flowering stage in the Spring…. Whereas, Thyme in Lithuania has the highest thymol levels during plant growth in July. (Full bloom stage). [22]

The Chemotype A (Alpha terpineol) in Thymus vulgaris, can survive in a hotter, drier, more arid climate than the other Chemotypes. Thus, the phenolic aspects of Chemotype A are to be credited for its ability to produce a higher carvacrol component in the essential oil. Whereas, the thymol dominance occurs in Thymus grown in wet areas. Keep in mind, knowing the difference of phenolic and non-phenolic oils will help you as an Aromatherapist, by knowing that phenols that grow in higher temperatures will vaporize much slower than non-phenolic oils that are grown in moist conditions. This information is helpful to know when vaporizing your oils for medicinal or aromatic purposes. Thus, Thymus vulgaris Chemotype A (Alpha terpineol) will be slower to vaporize than Thymus vulgaris Chemotype T (thymol) when you put it into the vaporizer or steamer.

On the other hand, studies show that Chemotypes T (thymol) & C (carvacrol) are phenolic oils that have a much higher inhibition zone when it comes to grasses germinating as opposed to the other Chemotypes, which are non-phenolic. This is important to know in the field production of plants used in the essential oil industry. The higher phenolic content of thymol & carvacrol allow for slower germination of grasses or weeds around the area of thyme commercial production, only on a temporary basis. [23]

For years, the essential oils found in plants were thought to just be substances that the plant was detoxing and really had no defined purpose. However, more recently, studies show that the volatile oils found in the leaves are present to protect the plant from moisture loss or as a defense mechanism. The genus, Thymus, along with Mentha, are the world's two most popular sources of thymol and carvacrol. These are the monoterpenoid phenols that make thyme and mint essential oils so sought after for their medicinal benefits.

I won't dive any further into the ORGANIC CHEMISTRY of Thyme, but should you be interested, doing your research into the INDIVIDUAL component properties and uses would truly enhance your knowledge of essential oils.

*"The art of medicine consists in amusing the patient
while nature cures the disease."*
~Voltaire

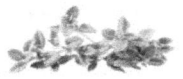

Components of Thyme Essential Oil

Now that you have read about the various Chemotypes of the Thymus vulgaris plant, I want to make mention of the components found in a couple of the Chemotypes. Each Chemotype will have a variety of constituents in varying quantities. I will give you an example of some of the healing components found in Thymus vulgaris CT thymol and CT carvacrol. I found this list of components in the book, 'Essential Oil Safety', written by Robert Tisserand/Rodney Young. The approximate percentages vary, but I have listed them from greater to lesser percentage, as listed in the 'Essential Oil Safety' book. Although, the book lists the actual approximate percentages of each and has a section describing the individual benefits of each component.

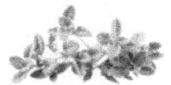

Thymus vulgaris CT thymol

Thymol
p-Cymene
Carvacrol
Gamma-Terpinene
Beta-Caryophyllene
Linalool
Alpha-Pinene
Alpha-Terpinene

[B.M. Lawrence, Progress in Essential Oils. (Perfumer & Flavorist 20 no. 3, 1995), 67. B.M. Lawrence, Progress in Essential Oils. (Perfumer & Flavorist 23 no. 1, 1998), 42-46. Source cited in Robert Tisserand and Rodney Young, Essential Oil Safety (Second Edition. United Kingdom: Churchill Livingstone Elsevier, 2014), 452-453.]

By comparing the CHEMOTYPE of the **ABOVE** Thyme variety with the CT component list **BELOW**, you can see how each CT can vary in component content, as well as, percentages of each constituent.

Thymus vulgaris CT Carvacrol

Carvacrol
p-Cymene
p-Terpinene
Thymol
Carvacrol methyl ether
Linalool
Alpha-Pinene
1,8 Cineole
Beta Myrcene
Alpha-Terpinene
 (Lawrence, 1989 p. 104-105) [24]

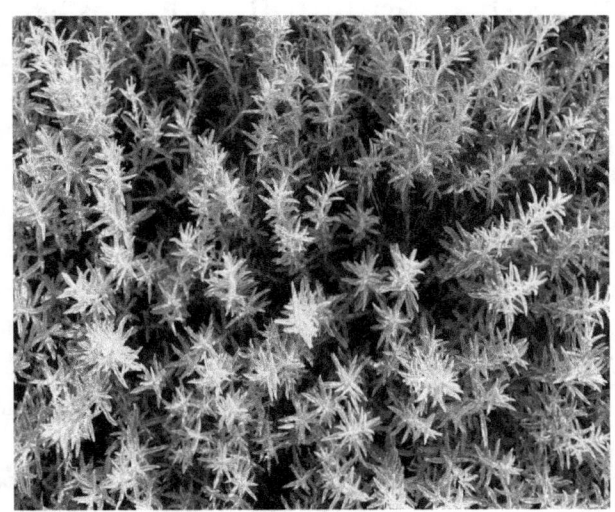

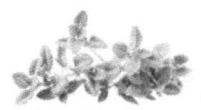

"It is more important to know what sort of person a disease has than to know what sort of disease a person has."
~Hippocrates (460-377 B.C.)

Types of Distillation Processes

Below are some of the common forms of distillation for essential oils. I realize this book is about Thyme Essential Oil, but I feel it is important to describe the various ways Thyme can be distilled. Please note that there are some specialty forms of distillation, as well as, outdated forms that are no longer used, that I have chosen not to mention herein.

Water Distillation

Plant material is brought to a boil in a container of water. Once the oils are released, the oil is separated from the water and bottled as essential oil. This same process can be done under a vacuum, of which the reduced pressure would allow for temps under 100 degrees Fahrenheit. This in turn, would allow tender, heat sensitive plants to survive the process and release their precious essential oils. Keep in mind, that any plant with a high rate of esters, should be steam distilled, instead. Esters tend to break down when exposed to such high heat factors. Floral waters are derived from water distillation. However, phenyl ethyl alcohol will dissolve in the hot water and must be distilled with an additional process. Ex: Rose Otto oil

Steam Distillation

Steam distillation is the most common form of distilling essential oils. This form of distillation is much like the water distillation process, except for one factor. This one difference is that the plant is not submerged in boiling water, but instead, the heat process is done beneath the container that holds the plant material and only the steam can pass through the material. This results in the essential oils being released from the leaves, bark, flowers, etc.... and traveling, along with the steam, through a tube that empties into a container. The water is drained off, resulting in hydrosols, while the oil is separated and sold as essential oils.

I suggest you go online and search for each of these distillation processes and then click 'Images' at the top and just look at various photographs of the distilling processes. Also check out the plethora of essential oil distillation videos on YouTube, as well as, the many distillation manufacturers.

Steam & Water Distillation Combo

This process is basically both water & steam distillation put together. The plant material is submerged in boiling water, while the steam is also allowed to penetrate and rise into the plant material. Thus, the steam and oils flow into the tube for collection, while the boiling water is also separated from the oils contained within once the proper time has elapsed for heating.

Hydro Diffusion

This type of distillation is the same as steam distillation, except it does have a higher yield and it is processed much quicker than traditional steam distillation processing. The only difference is the steam enters the holding chamber from the top, allowing the oil to drop through the bottom into an essential oil container.

Rectification

This is a process that is used to 'double distill' an oil when the oil has impurities remaining in it after the first distillation. Eucalyptus is sometimes double distilled and so is Thyme essential oil, when they take 'red thyme' and double distill it into 'white thyme'.

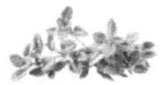

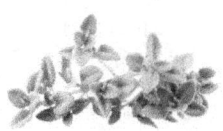

"I believe with all my heart and soul that God provided an answer for optimum body health. I believe the answers are found in the plants, their leaves, roots, flowers, bark, & stems, as well as, in the natural minerals found in the earth. I trust in the healing rays of the sunlight, in pure water, and in whole natural foods…. I trust natural substances when it comes to my WELLNESS rather than man-made synthetic versions. I feel that using the WHOLE plant gives SYNERGISTIC results that cannot be achieved by merely using ONE SYNTHETIC component and mixing it with substances that are not naturally found in the body."

~Karen Badea

Solvent Extraction Distillations

Solvent extraction methods involve using a solvent such as hexane, ethanol, methanol, and other substances such as petroleum ether. Benzene was once used widely until it was proven to be carcinogenic. This method of distillation is used for the more fragile flower material like jasmine, tuberose, etc. There are various forms of solvent extraction. I have mentioned a couple of the main forms below. I did not mention Enfleurage because of its prohibitive cost factor.

Maceration Distillation

This process involves delicate flowers being submerged into a container of animal fat that is heated to help the flowers release their oils into the fat. Once essential oils are released into the fat, the flower petals are removed and then the fat with the essential oils is bottled. This process is often used in the cosmetic industry and is a much more expensive process than steam distillation of essential oils.

Hypercritical Carbon Dioxide CO2 Extraction

Very recent form of extracting essential oils today. This process is becoming popular in the distillation industry. The process itself is done within a confined chamber and the pressure is altered over 200x that of normal environmental pressures. This substance creates a new form of 'magic' when it reaches 33 degrees Celsius. At this point, hypercritical CO2 becomes more of a solvent based substance, instead of any other expected form.

Hence, it's remarkable ability to extract essential oils from plant material. It is more expensive than steam distillation, but the results are instant, and the yield is far greater than other forms of distillation.

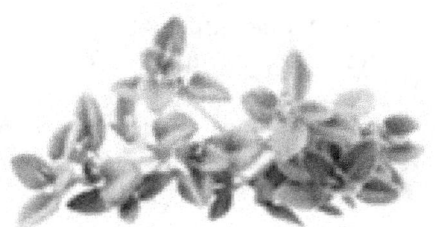

Expression Distillation
(Cold Pressing)

Expression distillation involved mechanical pressing to produce an essential oil. The perfect example is of citrus essential oils. There are basically three forms of Expression.

Ecuelle

This distillation method is used for citrus fruit peel oils. A machine has spikes and the citrus peels are punctured over and over with these spikes, causing the oils and pigments to run into a container. The container of oils and water are then separated, and the oils are bottled.

Machine Abrasion

This method of distilling essential oil is the one used by most commercial citrus essential oil distilleries. The citrus peels are loaded into a machine that cuts the peel on the fruit and then allows water to separate it from the fruit. The peel, with the oil content, is fed into a centrifugal separator, which then squeezes the oils out mechanically. The centrifugal separator works so fast. The waters and oils are then separated…

Sponge

This form of essential oil distillation involves a machine that will press, for example, citrus peels. These peels are first soaked in water and then put into a machine that presses the oils onto a sponge. The sponge is, in turn, squeezed into an essential oil container. [25]

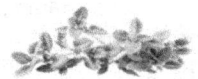

"I only wish that every soul on this planet would research the potency of plants."
~A Survivor of Lyme

Blending of Thyme Essential Oil

Thyme essential oil is often blended with Grapefruit, Lavender, Lemon, Rosemary, Pine, & Bergamot. A professional Aromatherapist can blend Thyme to make various recipes for bacterial diffusing, using Tea Tree, Ginger, Orange, Clove, Cinnamon, and, Basil. These blended oils are very effective in fighting bacterial pathogens and blending for respiratory issues. The blends can be used in a diffuser or rubbed on NEAT into the chest, or even used as air fresheners.

Keep in mind that it is a middle note and again, it will blend fantastically with lemon, lavender, pine, bergamot, grapefruit, eucalyptus, and rosemary. Moreover, using a blend that attains the synergistic formula of thymol, carvacrol, and eugenol components is very healing.

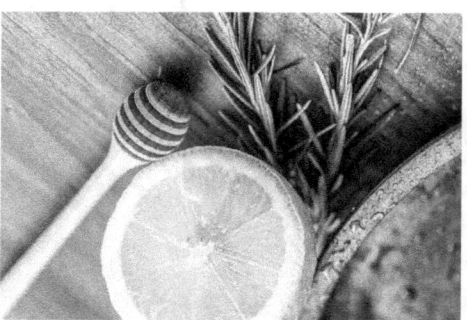

"I'm a big believer in what's called personalized medicine, which refers to customizing your health care to your specific needs based on your physiology, genetics, value system and unique conditions."
~David Agus

Polymorphism Traits of Thyme

One unique quality with Thymus vulgaris is its polymorphism traits. This trait means that the Thymus vulgaris plant can be either female or hermaphrodite. There is a difference in the size of the flowers between the female and the hermaphrodite plants. Female plants will have a minimized flower with no stem vs. the hermaphrodite, which has a little larger size flower and contains a stem. They have no need for a male plant. The female plants produce many more seeds than does the hermaphrodite plants. In addition, the female plants have much higher frequencies than do the hermaphrodite plants. The pollination of the process has been observed to be much easier with the female flowers. These flowers are pollinated in various seasons of the year, according to where they are growing in the world.

Thyme is known to grow best in well-drained soil and loves growing on sunny slopes that are full of rocks or can even be found near the Mediterranean Sea, growing on sand dunes near the water's edge.

Also, keep in mind, that Thyme plants have the genetic trait of producing various monoterpenes, resulting in different Chemotypes. The dominance factor of the monoterpene is found in the trichomes, which are found on the surface of the plant leaf. If you wish to learn further detail on the genetic traits (genotypes, phenotypes, alleles, etc....) then again, I suggest reading the book, 'Thyme...The genus Thymus' by Elisabeth Stahl-Biskup and Francisco Saez. [26]

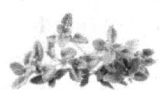

"Do not follow where the path may lead. Go, instead, where there is no path and leave a trail."
~Ralph Waldo Emerson

ORAC Value & Anti-Inflammatory Benefits

Thyme has an ORAC value (Oxygen radical absorbance capacity), which is a measurement of its antioxidant abilities. In comparison to oils like Clove, which has an ORAC value of over 1 million, Thyme has a minimum ORAC value at 15,960 units per 100 grams. However, it still has major antibacterial, antifungal, and other crucial benefit factors. One thing I did notice is that Thyme (dried or fresh) in plant form, has a higher ORAC value than thyme essential oil on the chart I've referenced herein. Keep in mind, Thyme is considered a 'hot' oil, therefore, it will burn when it touches your skin. This trait is one of the reasons that the oil needs to be handled with caution. Regardless, of its 'heat', it is a potent anti-inflammatory oil and considered a COX-2 inhibitor (COX-2 or cyclooxygenase-2 is an inflammation enzyme), which is a good trait for those suffering from inflammatory issues. Thyme essential oil will help to diminish inflammation in the body. At the same time, Thyme enhances PPAR receptors, activated by peroxisome proliferation, which, in turn, aids in suppressing COX-2 inflammatory enzymes, also. Thus, Thyme essential oil is a great oil used for general inflammatory issues and pain.

Thyme's COX-2 inhibitory element has even been known to reduce menstrual pain better than ibuprofen, according to a study done by Babel University of Medical Sciences in Iran. Those taking the 2% diluted capsule of thyme oil, along with a placebo instead of actual ibuprofen, had a remarkable improvement in pain. Studies stated, "In our study, Thymus vulgaris also was able to significantly reduce pain and spasm in our patients involved with dysmenorrhea, "remarkably ``. and also stated, As well as, "Unlike NSAIDs medications, Thymus vulgaris does not cause gastrointestinal complications and also relieves gastrointestinal disorders such as ulcers, indigestion, constipation, flatulence, and asthma". [27]

I also found the above study to state, "As the cost of treatments are significant for the patients and government and also some of them are partial and unsatisfactory, people increasingly turn to the methods of complementary and alternative medicine". [28]

For example, although there have been various methods recommended to cure dysmenorrhea (painful menstruation, abdominal cramping), but the side effects of these medications and the high cost of importing their raw materials encouraged us to investigate and compare the positive effect of Thymus vulgaris and ibuprofen on dysmenorrhea." [29]   People are starting to realize that the essential oils used medicinally do not have many of the harsh side effects that the pharma options often present.

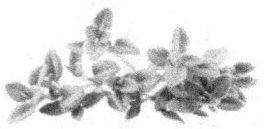

"With the growing recognition of the value of herbs, it is surely time to examine the professional therapeutic use of these herbs. There are profound changes happening in the American culture and herbal medicine, 'green medicine,' is playing an ever-increasing role in people's experience of this transformation."
~David Hoffman

Triple Blind Study

Below is a chart that will give you an idea on how
Thymus vulgaris rates against Placebo and Ibuprofen in
pain intensity studies.
Taken from Caspian Journal of Internal Medicine,
Thymus vulgaris vs. Ibuprofen vs. Placebo

Chart taken from: Thyme: Genus of Thymus, by
Elisabeth Stahl-Biskup and Francisco Saez. [30]

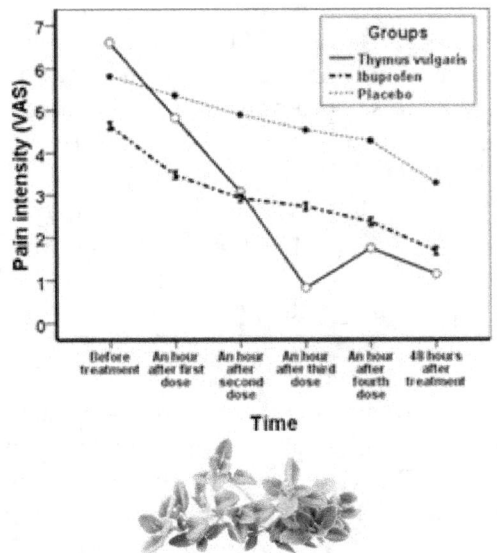

*"Nature does not hurry, yet everything is
accomplished."*
~Lao Tzu

Food Preservation Use of Thyme

Thyme's ability in the field of food preservation, is second to none. In fact, it has been proven that when used with mentha oil, the synergistic component factor is able to protect from food poisoning, naturally preserves food products, and also serves as an antifungal for food. [31] It has been proven to assist with staphylococcal food poisoning, as well as, pathogens such as Pseudomonas aeruginosa and Staphylococcus aureus. (MRSA), along with their biofilms and other Staphylococcus species. [32]

This precious oil is even said to be anti-parasitic. It can even treat intestinal parasites, like the hookworm. In addition, it has also been proven to combat Salmonella, Enterococcus, Shigella species, Pseudomonas, and Escherichia. [33] [34]
The components of carvacrol and thymol are the two 'heavy hitters' in the war against food pathogens. Thyme essential oil and Basil often work synergistically, as well, in preventing pathogens from growing on food products. [35]

Thyme essential oil has also been proven in studies to kill fungal Aspergillus forms. For example, in one study that I found in PubMed, the variety called, Zatoria multiflora Boiss. (Shirazi thyme) worked best on inhibiting growth of Aspergillus species. I'm not sure if this variety is readily available in the US due to government regulations. Shirazi thyme is grown mainly in the Pakistan, Iranian, and Afghanistan area of the world. It grows best in a dry arid environment. Its main components are the monoterpenes called thymol and carvacrol. It is a folk medicine for the Iranian natives. It has a long list of health benefits such as a diaphoretic, diuretic antiseptic, carminative, stimulant, anesthetic, analgesic antispasmodic, anti-inflammatory, antimicrobial, anti-viral, , and as an antioxidative agent, etc… [36] [37]

Another variety of Thyme that I found to be of interest is of Ethiopian origin and is called, Thymus schimperi. It has paramount antimicrobial abilities in studies where it was tested along with Cinnamomum zeylanicum. In fact, together they showed major antifungal and antibacterial qualities. [38]

Color of Thyme Essential Oil

As for the color of the different Thyme varieties of oil, they vary in color presentation. The distillation process is often repeated to get a different product. This entails the first distillation producing what some call Red Thyme, which has a Chemotype of thymol and is a much stronger crude form. The second distillation is the sweeter version, sometimes referred to as 'sweet thyme' and has the Chemotype of linalool. Of course, the CT itself can be determined by environment and growing conditions, as well. The red thyme oil is of a darker orange nature compared to the transparent light yellowish color of the sweet thyme (Thymus vulgaris, often known as 'common thyme'). [39]

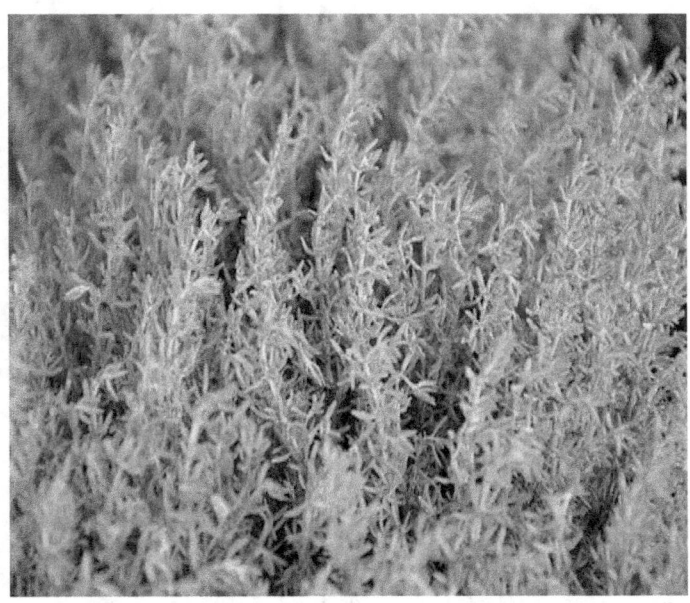

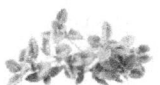

"Just as bees make honey from thyme, the strongest and driest of herbs, so do the wise profit from the most difficult of experiences."
~Plato

Benefits of Thyme Essential Oil

Antispasmodic - (suppresses muscle spasms)

Antirheumatic - (arthritic issues)

Antiseptic - (antimicrobial substance applied to living tissues)

Bactericidal - (Kills bacteria, whereas, IF something is bacteriostatic, it only stops bacteria from reproducing)

Bechic - (cough suppressant)

Cardiac - (heart related)

Carminative - (relieves flatulence)

Cicatrisant - (promotes skin regeneration)

Diuretic - (relieves water retention)

Emenagogue - (stimulates blood flow in the pelvic area and helps with menstrual issues)

Expectorant - (clears mucus from respiratory passages)

Hypertensive - (raises blood pressure) *See cautionary statement above

Insecticide - (kills/repels mosquitoes, fleas, lice, bed bugs, flies, beetles, moths)

Stimulant - (improves mental or physical functions)

Tonic and Vermifuge - (kills intestinal worms, helps with sour stomach, and the tonic restores one's' feeling of wellbeing.) Anti-Venomous - (Used to treat poison venom from animals or insect bites)

Health Conditions Treated With Thyme Essential Oil

Cancer
Acne & Toning Skin (Anti-Aging qualities)
Blood Pressure/Circulation
Bacterial Issues
Fungal Issues
Flatulence
Pain
Heart Health
Rheumatic Issues
Diuretic
Expectorant for Respiratory Issues (mucous)
Scars
Menstrual Issues/Body Odor
Oral Health (Listerine contained Thyme originally)
Gum Disease/Canker Sores/Bad Breath
Eliminates Toxins by stimulating urination
Uric Acid issues
Arthritis
Colds/Flus/Bronchitis
Asthma
Mood Enhancement
Digestive issues
Anti-Inflammatory effect on Ear Edema
Premature Aging/Baldness/Alopecia/Oxygenates
Scalp/Improves Blood Flow of Scalp
Atherosclerosis
Fatigue/Exhaustion
Regenerates capillary glands [40]
Coadjutant for Slimming
Myalgic Encephalomyelitis (ME)
Fatigue (CFS)
Multiple Sclerosis (MS) [41]

BREAST CANCER- (Known to kill Cancers due to the Terpenoids found in Thyme)

Here is a quote I found on Facebook posted on 'The Eden Prescription'....

"Thyme Essential Oil Kills 98% of Breast Cancer Cells in Vitro: The essential oil of the common herb thyme was discovered to kill 98% of human breast cancer cells (MCF-7) in vitro after 72 hours of treatment. This was at a concentration of just 0.05% (at 0.01%, thyme essential oil still killed >40% of the cells). Thyme was shown to be the most powerful at killing cancer cells of all the 10 herb and spice essential oils tested in this study and was also shown to potently kill lung cancer and prostate cancer cells. The next most potent essential oils for killing breast cancer cells in this study were from cinnamon, rose, chamomile and jasmine. In other studies, thyme has also shown activity against oral and ovarian cancer. Thyme is native to the Mediterranean and was heavily used by the ancient Greeks for food and various ceremonies. In fact, it was the Greeks who gave this herb the name "thyme." Thyme is used prolifically in Mediterranean cooking, which may help to explain the low cancer rates there. (Greek women have less than half the incidence of breast cancer compared to American women). Thyme, or its essential oil, has also been used in Ayurvedic and traditional medicine owing to its strong antioxidant, anti-bacterial, and antifungal (potently killing yeast such as Candida) properties. It makes a great addition to a healthy diet focused on organic fruits, vegetables and whole foods and can be used as a flavorful herb in cooking or simply prepared as a tea.
http://www.ncbi.nlm.nih.gov/pubmed/20657472" [42]
~Posted on
https://www.facebook.com/TheEdenPrescription/posts/641553945899640:0

ANTHRAX

In addition, to the above various quotes about using Thyme for medicinal purposes, I wanted to include these, as well. While reading an article from the website, http://younglivingessentialoils.com.au/thyme-essential-oil-aromatherapy/healing, Douglas Holt also stated, "According to Jean Valnet, M.D., thyme oil kills the anthrax bacillus, the typhoid bacillus, meningococcus, and the agent responsible for tuberculosis. The oil is also a stronger antiseptic than phenol, which was widely regarded for years as the ultimate germ killer." [43]

Moreover, Dr. Len Horowitz and Dr. Sebina DeVita wrote directions for using Thyme essential oil for treating Anthrax. Their directions were, "Thyme thymol (Thymus vulgaris CT thymol) and Melissa essential oil. — For Anthrax infection- Fill an empty capsule with about 12 or more drops of Thyme and 1 drop of Melissa essential oil. Take 3 caps a day for 10 days, rest 48 hours then start up again. Also rub these oils mixed with Massage Oil Base or V-6 Mixing Oil all over the body. Thyme 15 ml bottle." [44]

MULTIPLE HEALTH ISSUES

I also want to mention Holt's listing of Alzheimer's disease and hepatitis as benefiting from Thyme Essential Oil protocols, as well.

Douglas Holt wrote, "Daniel Penoel, M.D., recommends thyme CT linalool for tuberculosis, bronchitis, pneumonia, intestinal parasites, psoriasis, cystitis (bladder infection), nephritis (kidney infection), candida infections, and intestinal tract infections."
As for the beneficial attributes of the fragrance of Thyme oil, it is said to help manage fatigue, as well as, post illness exhaustion.

Douglas Holt recommended this protocol when using Thyme Essential Oil:

"Application: Dilute 1 part essential oil with 4 parts V-6 Vegetable Oil Complex or other pure vegetable oil; (1) apply 1-2 drops on location, (2) apply on chakras and/or Vita Flex points, (3) diffuse, or (4) take as a dietary supplement."

Additional protocols that Holt wrote about, include:
"At the first sign of a cold or flu, a drop of oil should be added to a tablespoon of honey and taken every half hour."

A drop or two of oil may also be sprinkled on a handkerchief or washcloth and inhaled directly as needed to treat respiratory or sinus conditions. In cases of serious respiratory conditions, systemic candidiasis, or local yeast infections, an enema or douche may be needed.

Thyme has been thought to increase intelligence and is said to prevent internal body fats from going rancid. Keep in mind the brain and the liver are the fat organs of our body. Apply to the feet reflex points for these organs, inhale deeply from the oil left on your hands, taking the oil molecules deep into the brain.

According to Carolyn Mein in her book, 'Releasing Emotional Patterns with Essential Oils', Thyme is the oil to restore security when we feel a lack of protection. Mix 2 –3 drops of oil combined with V6 mixing oil and apply about 2 inches above the belly button, rubbing in a clockwise circle. V6 mixing oil is a mixture of 7 food grade oils. It can be used as a carrier oil or to dilute a strong essential oil that one fears could cause skin irritation. Young Living sells this oil.)

Put 10-15 drops of thyme in a 1oz spritz bottle and spray mist the inside of your car, replacing those nasty commercial air fresheners.
Diffuse this oil in your office to ward off disease, increase intellectual levels, instill confidence and courage.

Thyme oil is good for battling infectious diseases, and has been used to combat the anthrax bacteria, diffusing as well as steam inhalation is effective to clean the air and enhance the immune system. Diffusing Thyme oil helps support normal breathing and relax the muscles of the respiratory tract.

Thyme it also is very supportive to your liver. It can strengthen your body's ability to produce glutathione levels that decrease with age. Dr Ray Sahelian states that glutathione deficiency contributes to oxidative stress, which plays a key role in aging and the worsening of many diseases including Alzheimer's disease, Parkinson's disease, liver disease, cystic fibrosis, sickle-cell anemia, HIV, AIDS, cancer, heart attack, and diabetes. He also says that glutathione is a powerful antioxidant found within every cell. Glutathione plays a role in nutrient metabolism, and regulation of cellular events (including gene expression, DNA and protein synthesis, cell growth, and immune response. Many "anti-aging" professionals work on getting glutathione levels up. Oral supplementations do not work because glutathione may not be able to cross the cell membrane."

[This article was written by Douglas Bruner Holt in the May 21, 2013 edition of, Young Living's 'Essential Oils' online site.] [45]

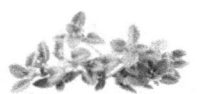

ANTIFUNGAL

As I mentioned previously, Thymus vulgaris is the most common thyme oil found in the western world, but there are some other very potent varieties that have been proven multiple times in medical efficacy. Thyme EO is known to be an antimicrobial and antifungal, among many other beneficial traits. In fact, its efficacy is so potent, that it has been proven to exceed even the antifungal medications purchased via a pharmaceutical prescription. For instance, a study in 2006, proved thyme to be among a few other essential oils as being one of the most potent for antifungal properties and even was proven to be more effective than the pharmaceutical prescription drug called Hexaconazole.

MRSA (Staphylococcus aureus)

In addition, thyme's efficacy against MRSA was also praised. [46] It is an extremely potent oil and should always be diluted with a carrier oil when used on the skin. So, not only is it considered a delicacy in the kitchen; it is revered as almost a sacred element in any medicine cabinet. One recipe that Aromatherapist use for combating MRSA is as follows:

3 drops of Thyme Essential Oil
3 drops of Oregano Essential Oil
2 drops of Rosemary Essential Oil

Blend together in a small glass container and add 10 drops of Extra Virgin Olive Oil. Use a dropper to fill a vegetable capsule. Consume the capsule with a meal.

Make sure to use all therapeutic 100% Pure Organic essential oils.

I bought a large clear glass cookie jar from Walmart and I keep my veggie caps in that jar for my essential oil protocols.

BACTERICIDAL SPRAY FOR HOME & AUTO

One very easy effective recipe I've used for combating MRSA bacteria (staph) at home and in my auto is this:

I buy a 6 oz spray bottle and add:

14 drops of Thyme Essential Oil
12 drops of Lemon Essential Oil
10 drops of Eucalyptus Essential Oil
8 drops of Rosemary Essential Oil
4 drops of Lemongrass Essential Oil

Place drops of essential oils in the bottle and then fill bottle with distilled water. This becomes your bacterial spray.

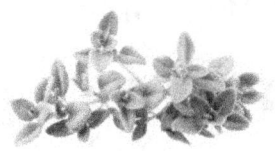

"Always laugh when you can. It is cheap medicine."
~Lord Byron

Compounding Components of Thyme With Other Plant Constituents for Healing

As quoted by a study entitled, 'Identification of volatile components in basil (Ocimum basilicum L.) and thyme leaves (Thymus vulgaris L.) and their antioxidant properties':

"In particular, eugenol, thymol, carvacrol and 4-allylphenol, found in basil and thyme, exhibited potent antioxidant activity, comparable to the known antioxidants, BHT and a-tocopherol." They went on to conclude, "Furthermore, ingestion of these aroma compounds may help to prevent in vivo oxidative damage, such as lipid peroxidation, which is associated with cancer, premature aging, atherosclerosis, and diabetes."

[Seung-Joo Lee a, Katumi Umano b, Takayuki Shibamoto c, Kwang-Geun Lee d,* Department of Food Science and Technology, Dongguk University, 3-26 Pil-dong, Chung-gu, Seoul 100-715, Republic of Korea b Takata Koryo Co. Ltd., 22-2 7-Chome, Tsukaguchi-Honmachi, Amagasaki, Hyogo-Pref. 661, Japan c Department of Environmental Toxicology, University of California, Davis, CA 95616, USA a Korea Food Research Institute, Seongnam-si, Republic of Korea. Received 4 May 2004; received in revised form 27 May 2004; accepted 27 May 2004] [47]

This is but one example of using compounding the components of Thyme with other constituents of other plants to heal. In addition to these fantastic components described herein above and, in the Thymus, vulgaris Chemotype section, Thyme is chocked full of Vitamin C and also contains vital Vitamin A, as well as other healing components. [48]

"A drop a day keeps the doctor away."
~ unknown

Using Thyme Essential Oil for Treating Gram Positive/Gram Negative Pathogens

One study that I found and is a paramount piece of information involving essential oils, in general, is this abstract quote,

"Gram-positive bacteria are known to be more susceptible to essential oils than Gram-negative bacteria.25,26 The finding that E. coli was least susceptible to 14 essential oils in this investigation is in accord with previous studies. The weak antibacterial activity against Gram-negative bacteria was ascribed to the presence of an outer membrane,27,28 which possessed hydrophilic polysaccharide chains as a barrier to hydrophobic essential oils. Accordingly, the high degree of susceptibility of H. influenzae was unexpected. One reason for this might be the hydrophobic nature of the outer membrane of H. influenzae forming rough colonies, in contrast to E. coli and Pseudomonas aeruginosa, which form smooth colonies.

Absence of cross-resistance between penicillin-susceptible and -resistant S. pneumoniae is due mainly to the different mechanism of action of essential oils compared with that of β-lactam antibiotics.29,30 Summarizing these results, we conclude that the antimicrobial action of essential oils by gaseous contact is most efficient when exposed at high vapor concentration for a short time. The results obtained in this investigation suggested that a maximal vapor level of 0.1–0.9 mg/L in air may suppress the growth of bacterial pathogens of respiratory infection."

[http://jac.oxfordjournals.org/content/47/5/565.long#ref-33 and written originally by J. Antimicrobe. Chemother. (2001) 47 (5): 565-573. doi: 10.1093/jac/47.5.565] [49]

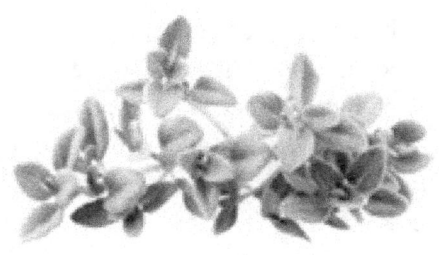

"Knowing yourself is the beginning of all wisdom."
~Aristotle

Spiritual & Psychological Benefits of Thyme Essential Oil

I've discussed some of the physical health benefits of this precious essential oil, and now I want to touch a bit on the spiritual and psychological benefits of using thyme essential oils.

Psychologically, thyme has been used for thousands of years as a mood enhancer. Roman soldiers were said to put thyme oil on them to make them feel less 'melancholy', as well as, thyme's ability to improve their cognitive abilities. Roman's often hung sprigs of thyme in rooms and used it in their pillows to help lift their mood. Roman soldiers would bathe in thyme to calm them and make them feel brave & ready for battle. An English knight's wife would embroider a sprig of thyme with a bee hovering over it into their husband's scarf. [50]

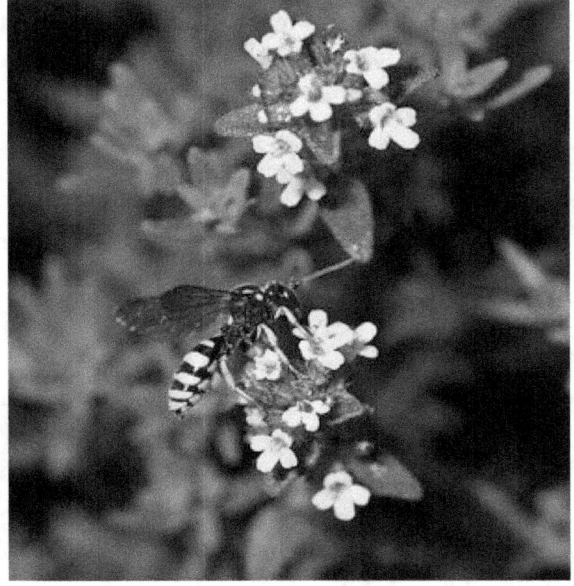

FYI: Thyme under your pillow is said to prevent nightmares while enhancing your dreams and psychic abilities.

Furthermore, a 2013 study proved the connection to the mood enhancement claims to be due to a neuromodulatory aspect from thyme's carvacrol component. [51]

This wonderful little perennial has been used for spiritual benefits for centuries upon centuries, as an incense. Thyme's aromatic nature is perfect for this use. The Greeks used it to burn in their holy temples and used it to instill elements of courage into the recipient. [52]

The chakras that thyme stimulates are the solar plexus and the heart chakra. Green is the chakra color that thyme is said to activate. [53]

Thyme was often used in ritual bathing before Spring events, representing 'washing off of the 'things of old' and 'bringing in the new'.

Aphrodite (Greek Goddess of Love/Fertility/Passion), Ares (Greek God of War), and Freya (Norse Goddess of War/Love/Sex) are said to sanction the use of thyme.

When using thyme in magic arenas, it is said to increase one's courage, strength, positive attitude, and luck with money.

It was believed by some in history to put a bundle of thyme into the casket of their loved ones would assist the soul to have a smoother transfer into the other dimension. Thyme tea was served to visitors of the family during mourning.

Burning dried thyme in the home after a disagreement is believed to dissipate the bad energies in the home. Thyme is said to balance relationship problems.

Some European traditions believe that faeries will be attracted to thyme patches in your garden. They also feel

that one can leave honey and thyme at the edge of the forest and the faeries will help you find something that you've lost.

It is believed that planting thyme in the garden will assure a financially prosperous life.

Thyme behind the ear or tied to your wrist is a sign of femininity and great for wearing when dating someone special.

Often thyme was/is used to encourage loyalty from a lover or spouse. It aids in purification rituals and if carried in your pocket or in a sachet around your neck or waist, it was believed to provide protection.

Thyme in the home is known to promote good health to all that live there.

Some say thyme is associated with the planet Venus and the element of water. Others say it is associated with Mars and associated with fire. Still others claim Venus and Air. I have no defined answer on this.

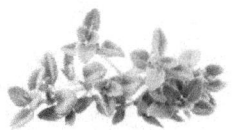

"The more you know, the more you know you don't know."
~Aristotle

Modalities of Using Thyme Essential Oil

Many will ask how thyme oil is best used for their health issues. Well, there are several ways to receive thyme's healing properties into your body.

Thyme essential oil can be:

- Diffused in the air via room diffusers
- Added to your bathwater
- Applied topically by diluting with a carrier oil
- Applied topically NEAT (directly on the skin without a carrier oil) Test skin to make sure oil does not irritate skin.
- Steam inhalation equipment
- Used in a nebulizer with professional guidance.
- Some can be used in food/drink recipes.
- Some can be used orally via gel caps with professional guidance. (Many professionals warn against oral use of thyme essential oil. (I take it internally via gel caps, but I do not recommend or promote this use).
- Used in skincare products (healing salves, etc.)
- Used in homemade soap recipes

Thyme essential oil is very healing to the respiratory system when used via steam inhalation but must be used with professional guidance. Remember, Thyme thujanol has been proven to kill Chlamydia species, including the airborne Chlamydia pneumoniae (CPN), that is often an opportune coinfection of other chronic issues, as well as Chlamydia T. [54]

Based on my experiences to date, I have found this to be a highly effective combination to kill Chlamydia Pneumoniae. Take oil blend along w/ 2400 mg. NAC

(N-Acetyl Cysteine) daily. This was found on
http://www.cpnhelp.org.

This skin protocol below uses thyme thujanol and was submitted by Dylan, Potential new protocol. Submitted by Dylan on Thu, 2012-03-22 02:17.

- **Lavender fine** - 1-4 drops (lavender fine alone can be used effectively to keep costs down)
- **Thyme thujanol** - 0-4 drops (very strong, seems to be synergistic with Lavender but may not be necessary to incorporate immediately)
- **German Chamomile** - 0-4 drops (doesn't appear to have direct anti-chlamydial action but it is highly anti-inflammatory and according to the literature it helps the body to eliminate bacterial toxins which seems to help with the die off reaction)

Mix in 15 ml (1/2 OZ) carrier oil (I found that Sesame or Jojoba both work well) applied topically once/day or as tolerated the mixture can be applied over most non-sensitive body parts to maximize surface area. Covering the skin afterwards with clothing or sheets helps to prevent evaporation and aids absorption."

(Lavender fine essential oil is distilled from plants that are grown at a high altitude. This variety is much more comprehensive lavender species that is preferred often over other varieties of lavender. Its great for skin spots and known to work well when skin needs soothing from sun burns. It is perfect to blend with Thyme CT thujanol)

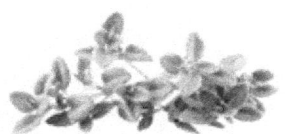

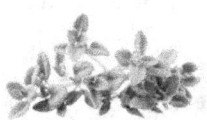

"I invite you to drink in the divine nectar of aromatic love and let it penetrate you in the deepest, most profound ways. Trust that the oils are working side-by-side to heal, regenerate, and teach you. The more you use them, the more they'll reveal their secrets to you".

~Elana Millman, Aromatherapy for Sensual Living: Essential Oils for the Ecstatic Soul

Historical Progression of Essential Oil Use

Thyme essential oil, along with other beneficial healing essential oils, used to be found only in a person's private homemade stash. Then it graduated to spas and being used by massage therapist for luxury purposes and onto health supplement stores. Later pharmacy stores started carrying supplements and essential oils and now, many medical doctors have their own 'in house' supplement shops and promote essential oils.

For instance, Lyme Literate MD's routinely recommend essential oils to their patients to combat pathogens and to help regulate the body. Essential oils, in general, are being shared by MLM representatives that teach the oils to their friends and families on a home party basis. I'm sure you are aware of at least two major MLM essential oil companies today. Not to mention, churches, which often share and teach natural health options to their members, as well as, Naturopath MD's, holistic nursing, hospitals, etc. and even the 'stay at home' Mom, whom value natural healing options for her family. Yes, essential oil knowledge is alive and doing well today.

Why? It's because essential oils have very little side effects. Whereas, antibiotics often have 'death' as a side effect. (I'd call that more than just a 'side effect', wouldn't you?) Also, for the fact that essential oils can go inside the fat tissues where pathogens often hideout. EO will kill deadly pathogens that harbor inside those fat cells away from main blood flow. Antibiotics cannot pass the fat cell or lipid barrier like essential oils do.

In addition, a very key benefit of using essential oils is the fact that they can pass through the blood brain barrier, as well. In addition, they can be taken orally, topically, nebulized, and via douche or enema. They are very versatile.

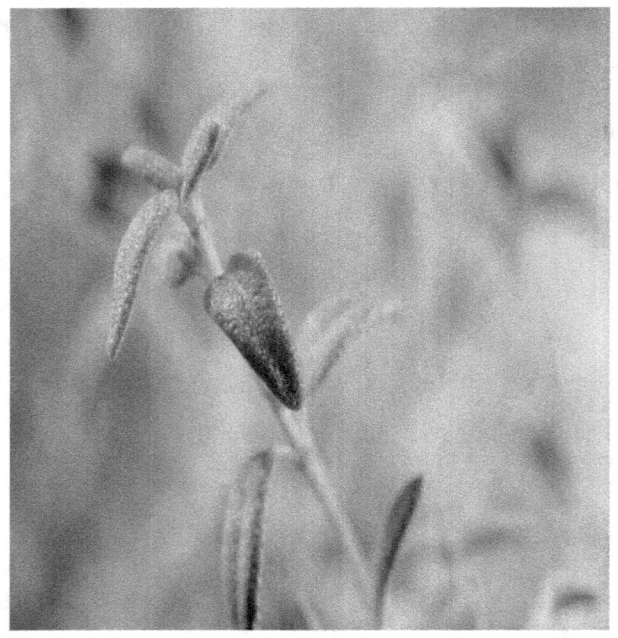

"One tradition I have with my friends is that when one of us gets married, we have a ton of fragrance oils and pretty bottles at the bachelorette party. Everyone puts a drop or two in a bottle for the bride and makes a wish, and the bride wears our creation on her wedding day."

~Jennifer Aniston

Commercial Thymol Industry

In addition to the flavor, medicinal, spice, topical use, perfume, and culinary benefits of thyme, there is a commercial industry built entirely to harvest the main healing component of thyme plants. That is a commercial industry that harvests thymol. However, many warn against using just the one healing component in wellness protocols. Why?

Because many experts feel that the entire plant has synergistic healing values that cannot be dismissed. Big pharma can sell a patented version of thymol, but cannot patent the entire plant, since it is a natural source and laws will not permit. Thus, profit potential is only based on the one constituent of producing thymol. Personally, if I had a choice, I'd try to use the entire plant. I suppose they feel that this works on the same principle of body, mind, spirit…. Using the whole plant, to work synergistically, would be my personal goal, as well.

As for the commercial distribution industry of the whole oil and thymol, finding a good distributor is paramount. There are many large commercial producers of thyme essential oil that allows the professional Aromatherapist to purchase wholesale direct without the 'middleman'.

One exceptional source that I plan on having access to, in my business, is Aromahead Institute's database of essential oil manufacturers. This is found at https://distillerdirectory.com/. [55] There is a first-time fee that is followed by a much lesser annual fee thereafter. While it is possible to 'google' for wholesale essential oil producers, it is very convenient to go to one location like the distiller directory that Aromahead Institute has built online.

Touring as much as possible of the worldwide essential oil producing facilities, will be on the top of my 'To Do List'. Becoming the best Aromatherapist entails learning the entire process from field to bottled product to customer application and their results.

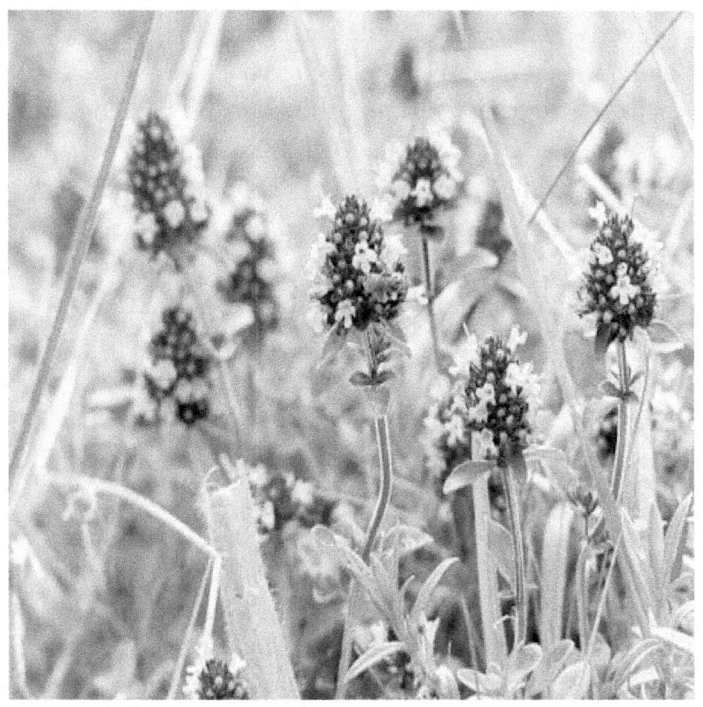

*"I've learned that people will forget what you said,
people will forget what you did, but people will never
forget how you made them feel."*
~ Maya Angelou

Safety Use of Thyme Essential Oil

Essential oils can be very dangerous if one isn't trained properly in safety precautions involving the proper usage and purification. Therefore, everyone needs to council with an Aromatherapist that knows the proper guidelines and knows how to read the GC/MS data. MLM essential oil salespeople are often not trained properly in the safety precautions of these medicinal oils. Although, there are some professional sales representatives that seek comprehensive training and are even Certified or Registered Aromatherapist. However, the inconsistency of training is a concern when it comes to safety using the oils. Keep in mind, that some of the large multi-level marketing essential oil companies offer a wide arrange of very valuable training for their representatives. It's up to the individual whether they pursue the available training.

Using essential oils for one's health is a very rewarding healing process. Although, the use of essential oils without proper guidance and training can lead to a dangerous situation. This caution is compared to when you purchase medications from a pharmacy, you trust your pharmacist to be aware of all safety issues in each chemical pharma drug. You would never use a drug without proper guidelines from a trained professional. The Aromatherapist is responsible in the same manner as the pharmacist in teaching the proper use of the essential oils that you chose to use.

Some of the cautionary issues when using thyme EO involves people with high blood pressure. Thyme essential oil can increase the blood circulation, thus, in turn, causing detrimental health issues. Although, thyme is used in culinary dishes and in teas, it is not recommended in the US to be taken internally. This is due to essential oil's cumulative strength in high concentration. Many Aromatherapist warn against internal use due to possible life-threatening scenarios with the heart, thyroid, blood pressure, body temperature, and lung functioning.

Regardless, many do take thyme internally and I am one of them. I also nebulize thyme essential oil, but do not promote this to others. Thyme should not be taken by pregnant women. It is a valuable medicinal oil but should be used wisely with supervision from a trained physician or Cert/Registered Aromatherapist. It is considered a warmer oil, so it does need to be highly diluted before applying. It can cause skin irritation in some people. [56]

Herein, I have mentioned the various Chemotypes of Thymus vulgaris, but I want to touch briefly on the safety of the major components found in thyme and their healing capacities.

I feel this is important for a better understanding of what organic constituents are, what they are capable of treating, and the safety issues involved in various scenarios when using essential oils in general.

Safety is paramount in all instances and knowing where to turn to get the best professional advice is of utmost importance. The therapeutic value of any oil is determined by the organic components found in that oil and the percentages of constituent dominance. By sending your oils to a GC/MS lab where they have the spectrometry equipment to analyze your oil, this is the only way to be totally safe and know exactly what your oil contains. If you purchase your essential oils from a large distributor, they usually always furnish the GC/MS data reports for each oil. If not, you need to find a distributor that does openly offer them. Your liability factor can hinge on these data forms. They are vital to your client's health and also to running a good solid practice.

However, I also use a very valuable tool that I've just added to my library of essential oil books. It is a book that I turn to when deciding the safety value and toxicity level of an oil. The book is entitled, 'Essential Oil Safety' and is a large hardback book written by Robert Trissand and Rodney Young. [57] This is a 'must have' book for the professional Aromatherapist. It contains the general chemical analysis of many oils and is an authority on essential oil safety. This book breaks down the average percentages of components in various essential oils and has a section that describes the toxicity levels of each major component. Although, it does not have every variety of plant oil, it does carry the most popular and their Chemotypes. Robert Tisserand is leading authority and independent expert in the essential oil industry. He was publisher and editor of the industry's leading trade publication, The International Journal of Aromatherapy. Mr. Tisserand's website is very informative and offers additional paid training courses: http://roberttisserand.com/. [58] His 'Essential Oil Safety' book lists various thyme varieties and Chemotypes.

Always be cognitive to the fact that distributors often adulterate essential oils to gain a maximum profit. The substances mixed with the pure oils are often synthetic. Many distributors will stock in their inventory various single synthetic components and add these components to the pure oils, therefore diluting the healing potential of the oil and causing a synthetic chemical to be consumed in the body. It is very important to order from reputable sources and to require the GC/MS sheets to verify the purity factor of the oils you will be using and selling to customers.

Distributors are very wise when it comes to using synthetics that will be able to pass the 'purity smell test'. GC/MS data reports are paramount to cover you legally should any adulteration issues arise with customers concerning the oils you provide to them.

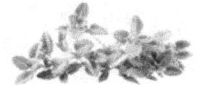

ADDITIONAL ESSENTIAL OILS THAT BLEND WELL WITH THYME

1. GRAPEFRUIT ESSENTIAL OIL
2. LEMON ESSENTIAL OIL
3. ROSEMARY
4. PINE
5. LAVENDER
6. BERGAMONT
7. OREGANO
8. MELALEUCA (TEA TREE)

These blended scents are especially clean and aromatic.

More importantly, they compound healing components

when treating various health issues.

THYME ESSENTIAL OIL can be diluted with coconut oil by adding 1-2 drops to 1 Tsp of Coconut Oil and this can be used topically for various skin issues. I often add TEA TREE ESSENTIAL OIL & LEMON ESSENTIAL OIL to my THYME ESSENTIAL OIL in 2 TBSP COCONUT OIL. I mix this and keep it in a tiny purse size salve container.

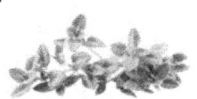

INTERNALLY, I take what is referred to as 'MY LYME AMMO' when I'm not feeling well. Especially around the FULL or NEW MOON times of the month. I must admit, my Lyme symptoms are sometimes overwhelming.
I drop the oils into a size '00' veggie capsules. YOU MUST CONSULT YOUR LYME MD ON THIS FIRST!!!

MY LYME AMMO
I USE FOR MY PERSONAL HEALING JOURNEY

1. 2 DROPS THYME (PLANT THERAPY)
2. 2 DROPS FRANKINCENSE (PLANT THERAPY)
3. 6 DROPS OF OREGANO (86% CARVACROL)(ZANE HELLAS)
4. 12 DROPS 'THIEVE'S (YL) OR GERM FIGHTER (PLANT THERAPY)

Drop into size '00' veggie capsule. Depending on the severity of my symptoms, I take one per day, but when I was really suffering from my symptoms, I took 1 every 6 hours. I regulated my dosage according to the 'herxing'. (A Herxheimer refers to the symptoms one suffers from die-off of pathogens). A Lymies first date with 'herxing' is a nightmare. A nightmare that never stops sometimes for years until the pathogens are minimized and the body has detoxed properly. (NOT a fun place to visit).

"Life isn't about finding yourself. Life is about creating yourself."
~ George Bernard Shaw

Thyme Varieties

Although, we have mentioned Thymus vulgaris (Common thyme) and some other Middle Eastern and European species, I wanted to put a list of some of the more popular thyme species that can be bought in the US. Their floral colors vary in color ranges from blue-violet, lilac, mauve, pink, and white flowers. The leaves of these species can vary in green intensities, and as silver or golden. When the leaves are crushed between your fingers, the aroma is splendid. Each variety looks differently and is often of a different size. While some are like a low-lying bush, others grow flat like a living carpet. They love rocky soil and dry arid climates. I have listed a chart of a few of the more popular varieties.

Thyme (borneol)	Moroccan thyme	*Thymus satureioides*	Morocco
Thyme (geraniol)		*Thymus vulgaris*	France
Thyme (lemon)	Lemon Thyme	*Thymus x citriodorus*	Mediterranean
Thyme (limonene)		*Thymus vulgaris*	Spain
		Thymus serpyllum	
Thyme (linalool	Sweet Thyme	*Thymus vulgaris*	France
		Thymus zygis	
Thyme (spike)	Spiked thyme	*Thymbra spicata*	Europe
Thyme (thujanol		*Thymus vulgaris*	France
Thyme (thymol		*Thymus vulgaris*	France
		Thymus zygis	
Thyme (carvacrol		*Thymus vulgaris*	France
		Thymus zygis	
Thyme (thymol/c arvacrol)		*Thymus serpyllum*	Europe
		Thymus zygis	

Culinary Thyme

Caraway Thyme	*Thymus herba barona*
English Thyme	*Thymus vulgaris*
'French' Thyme	*Thymus vulgaris*
'Golden Lemon' Thyme	*Thymus citriodorus*
Grey Hill Lemon Thyme	*Thymus vulgaris*
Hi-Ho Silver Thyme	*Thymus argenteus*
Italian Oregano Thyme	*Thymus nummularius (many others)*
Juniper Thyme	*Thymus leucotrichus*
'Minus' Thyme	*Thymus praecox 'Minus'*
'Mother of Thyme'	*Thymus serpyllum*
Orange Balsam Thyme	*Thymus vulgaris*
Pennsylvania Dutch Tea Thyme	*Thymus pulegioides*

Thyme Caveats

- Be cautious when using thyme essential oil!
- Be aware that natural products DO NOT always mean they are 'healthy'
- American & British Aromatherapy teaches to NOT take thyme internally. They feel that thyme EO can harm the liver, heart, lungs, and even stimulate the thyroid, resulting in issues if one has a hyperthyroid issue. However, French and other foreign traditions embrace taking Thyme EO supplementation, orally, as I do.
- Do not use thyme essential oil on children. (Although, some Aromatherapist use thyme linalool on children. It is the 'white thyme 'and it isn't as strong as 'red thyme'.)
- Do not use thyme EO on people with high blood pressure.
- Avoid using thyme EO during pregnancy due to menstrual stimulation.
- Test thyme EO on skin before using a large amount.
- Thyme EO is a mucous membrane irritant.
- Maximum dilution should be: adults 1%.
- Do not use if you have allergies to rosemary or mint essential oils [59]
- BEWARE: 'RED THYME' is often TOTALLY ADULTERATED, in other words, TOTALLY SYNTHETIC!!! Hence, instead buy, '100% THERAPEUTIC ORGANIC' ESSENTIAL OILS ONLY!' [60]

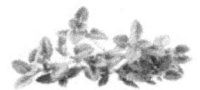

Drug Interactions with Thyme Essential Oil

- Thyme essential oil should not be used with persons taking anticoagulants.
- Do not use thyme essential oil If you are having/had recent MAJOR SURGERY
- Do not use thyme EO If you have a PEPTIC ULCER
- Do not use thyme EO If you have HEMOPHILIA
- Do not use thyme EO If you have a BLEEDING DISORDER [61]

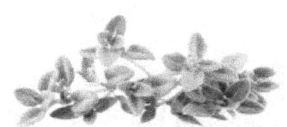

"It's what you learn after you know it all that counts."
~John Wooden

BONUS SECTION ONE

Aromatherapy Education & Professional Resources

In this section, I want to mention some phenomenal resources that every Aromatherapist should have in their 'tool bag'. I also want to share a bit about the requirements to become a Certified or Registered Aromatherapist. The essential oil revolution is here. The internet holds such vast amounts of information about TRUTH in MEDICINE. This information base was never available to society, ever in history, until the past few decades. We are living in a great time to be able to have access to such a huge collective bank of knowledge around the world. Yet, this 'bank of free knowledge' while expanding progression is also a threat to the 'big boys' that control the chemical medical industry. So, learn, teach, & share all that you know about natural medicines, plants, and essential oils because one day, the 'money boys' could influence lawmakers to pass laws that forbid our current constitutional rights of free speech or even hinder our access to healthy plants and oils. As we all know, these 'good old boys have deep pockets.

'Any who'…Aromatherapy is THRIVING today! Technology is, indeed, assisting the expansion of global growth & knowledge of the essential oil industry. Medicinal essential oils are meaningful and life altering substances

Many dedicated Aromatherapist have gotten into the field after facing tragic health issues themselves. Illness is what coaxed me to use the essential oils. I will have the 'rest of the story' in my Lyme story that I will publish in the latter part of 2019.

I am so blessed to be open minded enough to take the leap of faith and use the oils for the first time. I hope this little bonus section will encourage you to seek additional information on becoming a Certified or Registered Aromatherapist.

I shared with you earlier that I decided on Aromahead Institute to attain my Certified Aromatherapist education. I feel very pleased to be a graduate of this aromatherapy program.

There are so many things to learn about essential oils. I've taken online chemistry courses, read a ton of books on organic chemistry of essential oils, as well as completed chemistry & premed biology courses at the university level as part of my degree. I'm amazed at the medicinal uses of these components found in the oils...

So, in the spirit of encouraging the continued learning experiences for all new Aromatherapist, I want to mention Aromahead Institute's database of individual component information. The link to this is https://components.aromahead.com/.

This, too, has a one-time initial fee that is followed annually by a much lesser fee. [62]   This database is something that I plan on taking advantage of in my own practice. I wanted to share this online component database with those needing a quick, convenient, and thorough resource to help them better assist their clients.

One very important factor in the ongoing educational process of a professional Aromatherapist is to always stay abreast of the latest information in the essential oil industry. A very organized and convenient way of doing this is to be a member of the National Association of Holistic Aromatherapy (NAHA) and/or the Alliance of International Aromatherapists (AIA).

If one wants to attain the highest level of education in Aromatherapy, of course, becoming a Registered Aromatherapist is possible by taking advanced courses, beyond the Certification curriculum, from a NAHA and AIA approved school. Once the advanced courses are completed, then one can apply to take the test given by The Aromatherapy Registration Council.

Although there are no mandatory government regulations to be an Aromatherapist, attaining the standards of the above-mentioned Aromatherapy organizations, is the highest level of education in Aromatherapy that one can reach in the Aromatherapy industry, within the US.

Moreover, as for the beginnings of my journey into essential oils, I thought it best to start my educational journey with becoming a Certified Aromatherapist. This also included learning the basics of organic chemistry. The chemistry of the oils is paramount in being able to choose the proper oil for the health condition that is being treated. I went to both essential oil association sites and looked at the schools that were approved by both associations and after investigating all applicable school programs, I chose Aromahead Institute. I am a proud graduate of Aromahead Institute, based in Florida. Wow, what a fantastic interactive online course they offer. I was very pleased. They even offer monthly payment plans for those not wanting to pay one lump sum.

One can learn the advanced international clinical benefits from a French Aromatherapist, in France, after completing the advanced course with Aromahead University. French clinical protocols include internal use of the essential oils. The use of essential oils is accepted in mainstream medicine in France. They use them orally, as well as, topically and aromatically.

Enhancing one's expertise to the level of being able to instantly recognize individual components, both synthetic and natural, by sniffing the oils alone is a talent that most all Aromatherapist hope to accomplish... (Similar to a professional wine connoisseur being able to isolate ingredients in a sample of wine).

I take the oils myself, internally, every day for my health issues, but cannot recommend this to my clients per NAHA standards in the US. Therefore, I am only sharing my personal experiences, herein. I look forward to expanding my education and hopefully doing a short internship in France to better understand their philosophy on medicinal essential oils.

Great Britain also uses the oils therapeutically, although they do not use them internally. I knew that the US organizations promoted only topical, message, compress, vapor and inhalation use of these oils. This doesn't mean that some people do not ingest essential oils in their medicinal protocol. MANY people do and I'm one of them. This only means that an Aromatherapist cannot professionally suggest this to their clients in the US by organizational standards. You are free to treat as you choose.

I must remind you to consult your medical professional about ingestion before you take any essential oil protocols. (Keep in mind that in America, the 'powers that be' have been accused of suppressing healing information on the oils.) Some think that they, perhaps, do not want ingestion to be promoted, since it would compete with corporate 'big pharma' profits. So, essential oil associations try to stay 'under the radar' of 'big brother' by just supporting aromatic and topical uses of the oils.

Most recently, the FDA came down on two of the larger essential oil companies for promoting the essential oils to heal specific health issues. The thousands of representatives had to be retrained to comply to the new FDA complaints and guidelines. Many feels this is just another way to protect the 'pharma boys' from losing profits because of the 'awakening' that is going on in this country, when it comes to natural and alternative healing options. Some are saying that our 'freedom of speech' will be 'hit' next and that, eventually, we won't be able to write about them either. We live in a very different world today. One where chemicals override nature, 'crazy overrides logic, profit overrides truth in medicine, etc.... Yet, due to the profound chemical side effects of pharma, people are starting to seek natural options for medicine. To the corporations, it's all about the money. Thank goodness, for now, they cannot patent nature. However, they do take individual components and synthesis them in order to patent their products. Sadly, I do expect them to eventually try to limit our access to the essential oils by deeming them 'unsafe'. This in turn, puts them as the 'gatekeeper in charge' of the plants. Seeing $$$ signs yet?

The saddest part of becoming an Aromatherapist and wanting to help 'cure' or 'heal' clients, is finding out, for the first time, the true hidden politics of the 'system'. Fore, in the USA, the system is geared to treating symptoms only. Anyone that claims 'healing' or 'cures' can be arrested. The 'matrix' loves to instill 'fear' into society when they are losing profits.

Nonetheless, in my learning process, I have filled my bookshelves with Essential Oil information. One of my resources for Thyme production processing is a FREE pdf manual that I found online.

It is a very comprehensive Thyme growing manual compiled by Directorate Plant Production in collaboration with members of SAEOPA and KARWIL Consultancy and published by:

Directorate Agricultural Information Services
Department of Agriculture, Forestry and Fisheries
Private Bag X144, Pretoria, 0001 South Africa
http://www.genesisseeds.com/organicseed/herbs/pdf/Ess
OilsThyme.pdf [63]

As for finding wholesale sources of essential oils, this task is difficult for the new Aromatherapist. Hence, my first resource would be to mention Aromahead's Distillery Directory, that I mentioned previously. It is quite a task to find wholesale essential oil producers in the US, due to the fact that oils are sold to large brokerage houses. Corporations then purchase, in bulk, leading to many companies 'enhancing' their oils with diluted carrier oils and other synthetic components that 'fluff' their profits and diminish your end oil quality. In other words, many oils on the market are diluted before they reach your hands. As a professional, it is wise to order direct from the small organic distillers. Most will be found outside the US.

I did, however, find a Minnesota company, Veriditas Botanicals Essential Oils, that is a member of the Provence, France coop and operates by the European standards of ECOCERT, the French certification association. They purchase from only small USDA Certified organic farmers around the world and do not deal with brokerage houses. This company does not sell to individual customers like the large MLM's. Instead, they distribute via their retailers. I noticed that one of their top customers is a famous natural health school university. They do carry thyme as part of the oils in their repertoire. Finding good reputable sources as direct as possible to the original source, (preferably the distiller) is the goal. Here is the website of the above mentioned: http://veriditasbotanicals.com/about-us/purity-integrity/ . [64]

Although, this is but one US supplier, many Aromatherapist choose to buy direct from the grower. A professional Aromatherapist will always have the ongoing task of constantly being aware of the latest best sources worldwide for their oil supplies. However, I do want to 'dabble' a bit into the 'artisan' side of distilling my own oils. So, I'm purchasing my own personal copper essential oil distilling equipment. I've found a copper essential oil distillery equipment manufacturer in Portugal and look forward to making my own essential oils for my personal use and to experiment with the distillation production process, on a small level.

I'm looking forward to producing my own thyme essential oil from my own dried thyme, grown in my own herb garden. Of course, this will be in a small quantity just for personal use and done for the educational knowledge. Keep in mind, there are many distillation equipment manufacturers. One of my friends owns a stainless-steel version that he uses to distill his own personal oils. There are even a few US winery locations that are curiously dabbling as artisan essential oil distillers.

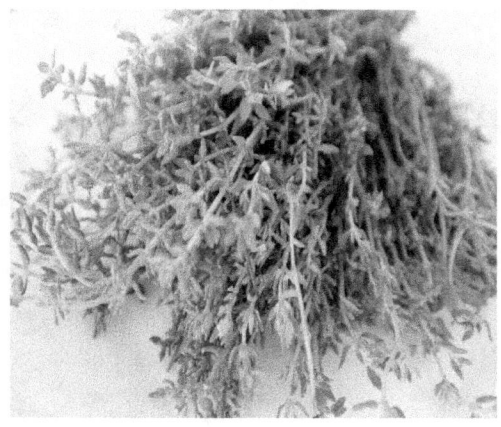

"Medicine rests upon four pillars - philosophy,
astronomy, alchemy, and ethics."
~Paracelsus

GLOBAL ESSENTIAL OIL INDUSTRY ASSOCIATIONS/WEBSITES

National Association Holistic Aromatherapy - naha.org

United States Lavender Association - www.uslavender.org

Essential Oil Association (EOA) -
www.facebook.com/pages/category/Health-Beauty/Essential-Oil-Association-134412120467198/

www.fda.gov/cosmetics/cosmetic-products/aromatherapy

Research Institute for Fragrance Materials -
https://www.rifm.org/

ThomasNet- https://www.thomasnet.com/products/essential-oils-54772405-1.html

American Essential Oil Trade Assoc.
https://www.facebook.com/AEOTA.US/

Int'l Trade Center -
http://www.intracen.org/itc/sectors/essential-oils/

https://www.perfumerflavorist.com/fragrance/application/mult iuse/Standards-and-Specifications-Essential-Oil-Association-of-the-USA-Inc-377810571.htm

(BRITISH EO ASSOC)…http://www.beoa.co.uk/
E.F.E.O. European Federation of Essential Oils …
efeo@wga-hh.de

USA - Fragrance Creators Association (former IFRA North America)

FRANCE CIHEF - Comité Interprofessionnel des Huiles Essentielles Françaises

FRANCE - SNIAA - Syndicat National des Industries Aromatiques Alimentaires, Aromatic Raw Materials Branch

GERMANY DVAI - Deutscher Verband der Aromenindustrie e.V.

GERMANY- DVRH - Deutscher Verband der Riechstoff-Hersteller e.V.

GERMANY -VDC - Drogen- und Chemikalienverein e.V.

SPAIN - - AILIMPO - Asociación Interprofesional de Limón y Pomelo

I also wanted to take the time to mention some free educational sites, in addition to Essential Oil University, of which, I mentioned previously. These are educational online sites that would cost nothing, but your time.

1.University of Minnesota Center for Spirituality & Healing –
http://www.csh.umn.edu/free-online-learning-modules/index.htm

2.Technical University of Madrid –
http://ocw.upm.es/ingenieria-agroforestal/industrial-utilization-of-medicinal-and-aromatic-plants

3. Aromahead University, Introduction to Essential Oils - http://aromahead.com/courses/online/introduction-to-essential-oils

4. Easy Courses Portal (Aromatherapy Free Course) - http://www.easycoursesportal.com/aromatherapy/course/Less-1.htm

The serious Aromatherapist will want to be a member of the Aromatherapy trade organizations. Two very important ones are:
NAHA – National Association Holistic Aromatherapist
AIA – Association International Aromatherapist

In the links below, you will find the schools that NAHA and AIA have approved for attaining your Certification as an Aromatherapist.
https://naha.org/index.php/education/approved-schools/

http://www.alliance-aromatherapists.org/education/aromatherapy-schools/

ARC is the Aromatherapy Registration Council that oversees the testing and qualifications for Registered Aromatherapist.
http://aromatherapycouncil.org/

Remember, the trade organizations offer the annual conferences that are the professional Aromatherapists best way of keeping up to date with the latest info in the industry. One can learn about the conferences by checking the NAHA and AIA websites for dates/time. They are often moved geographically each year within the US and also the international circuit. Many offer tours of local distillation plants and other aromatherapy interest. Not to mention, the access to networking with likeminded people. These organizations offer tons of annual training opportunities.

Another source for self-education would be the plethora of essential oils and aromatherapy books found on Amazon. Essential oils and Aromatherapy are such booming industries that it isn't difficult to self-educate these days. In fact, the smallest of local libraries usually always have books on essential oils and aromatherapy.

Not to mention, the large multi-level marketing companies that sell essential oils. They have representatives that are usually in your local area. These representatives are always eager to teach and train you or small groups on essential oils and their many benefits. This could be a learning experience for you and your friends. These company representatives refer to their training sessions as 'classes' instead of 'home parties' like many MLM's have done in the past. Regardless, they will hold classes in your home, at your

church, or at a local meeting source. The two largest MLM essential oil companies are Young Living (the oldest) and doTERRA, growing in leaps and bounds. There are tons of essential oil distributors. I order often from Plant Therapy. I only purchase THERAPEUTIC ORGANIC essential oils.

If you are not already an Aromatherapist, I encourage you to research the industry in depth. I feel every family should have a well-trained Certified Aromatherapist to consult with in times of need. I'm a big supporter for each family having an inventory of healing essential oils in their medicine cabinet. I have seen firsthand what the oils have done for my wellness factor. As I've said previously, I owe my life to them. I hope you will follow through and find the urgency to educate yourself in Aromatherapy protocols.

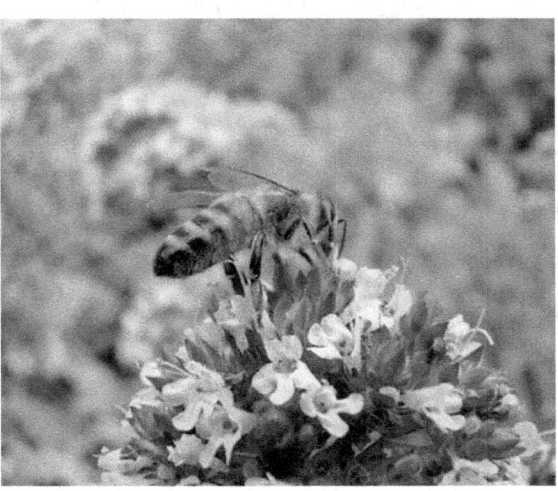

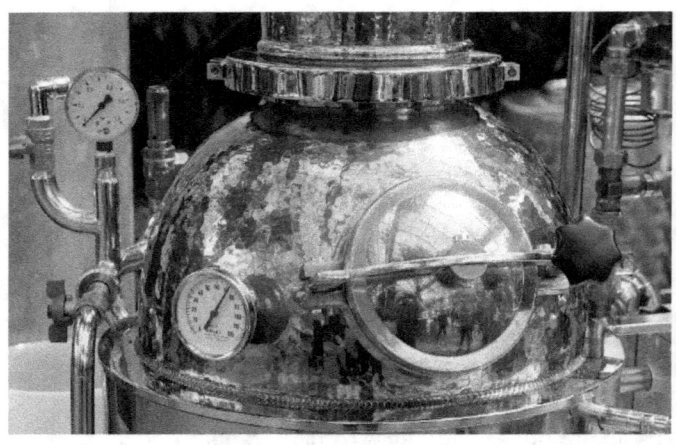

MY NEBULIZER USE OF THYME:

Yes, I am guilty. I do use thyme essential oil in my nebulizer. I am not recommending this to you unless you ask your physician. Myself, I add about 2 tbsp of distilled water to a glass container and 1 drop of thyme essential oil. I MADE SURE THE NEBULIZER CONTAINER WAS GLASS!!! I purchased my nebulizer glass container on Amazon and they shipped it from Asia. I ordered it as a replacement container for a diffuser/nebulizer. The tubing fit perfect on the glass container. It is paramount to use glass only, because the plastic cup that comes on the nebulizer, will degrade if oils are used in it. (Hmmm…Might this be 'why' they put PLASTIC cups on the nebulizers you purchase in this country? Could it be that they don't want us using OILS?)

'Anywho',(Ouch, that's my Southern slang again.)…. here is what I used in my own nebulizer when my lungs were having such issues. As I mentioned, I was diagnosed with CPN after asking my local family doctor, of 20+ years, to test me. In fact, the nurse practitioner told me that I was the FIRST in my local hospital to ever be tested for CPN. When I asked for the test, they knew not the 'politics' behind it. (I did but they did not… However, I think they quickly learned.)

Regardless, I was positive, and I went on to find a doctor that was honest and saved my life. My doc's explanation of the test results was, "Everyone, even I, have CPN. This isn't anything to worry about." I knew differently and I quietly thanked him and left the office with my own copy of the test results. I went immediately to Tennessee to a physician that a friend in TN had told me about. I also simultaneously researched everything I could find on CPN, including the physicians that studied this.

Luckily, the TN doc that treated me for CPN with PULSING antibiotics for a year was best friends with one of those professor MD's…. GOD WAS WATCHING OVER ME! Thank God, I was able to find this 'loophole' because the same antibiotics he treated me with for CPN were also the same used to treat Lyme. (I had an appointment with my Lyme Literate MD, but it was 6 months away. I would have died otherwise.) I was in a frenzy to learn the natural treatments and politics behind all that I was facing, while struggling to exist, all at the same time. I knew I had ONLY ME to figure it out and figure it out QUICK!!.

The 'powers that be' had just slapped this CPN doc's hand' for treating people for CPN and he had to stop treating. I was his last patient that he treated for CPN. He first denied me and then walked out of the room and back in and asked, "Do you realize this treatment is 1 year and can you commit to it? I said, "Yes" and he warmed up and agreed to help me. I was so sick I didn't think I'd live to make the trip back home to Kentucky. He was in fear of his license, but saw I was seriously dying. That man had a heart!!! Let me tell ya!!!

Thank goodness I quickly learned about the potency of Thyme in lab studies against CPN. Sadly, I had to lead my own healing strategies. I had no one that would help in my home state. They all rejected me after testing positive for Lyme, CPN, etc... I scared them. You see, a medical doctor takes a chance on losing their license for treating a Lyme patient after 28 days. So, they want you 'out of their hair' immediately. If you find yourself on the floor looking up and fighting pathogens that you've never heard of, well, sister Kate, you better be prepared to research and treat naturally, because otherwise, sweetheart, you are a 'dead duck'.

The 'politics' around Lyme is very mysterious and the system absolutely refuses to admit there is CHRONIC LYME spreading throughout the US in untold numbers each year. EVERYONE IS 'in bed' with everyone else when it comes to these organizations and associations…. You are ON YOUR OWN!! They turn a blind eye.

Some say it's due to a secret military experiment, but I don't know anything about that. I do recommend reading 'LAB 257' if you are interested in this subject.

Geeezzzz, the young ER doc in a large university hospital in my state, walked out of the room when I requested Lyme testing for the heart issues and seizures I was having…He looked up at me, smiled, and said, "There is no Lyme in KY" and walked out. The nurse came in and released me to go home in that bad of a health situation. I was appalled. UNBELIEVABLE!!

They were going to let me die rather than deal with 'Lyme'. I ended up finding out that I had not only Lyme but several deadly coinfections. Luckily, I found nature to be on my side and I tested myself via an online lab that used LabCorp and my docs had to accept the results, but they still didn't treat me. I'll explain further in my future Lyme story.

Indeed, I thank GOD for thyme essential oil and the nebulizer that a local doc prescribed for me, whom wasn't even my regular family doc. I found a doc that was rejected by our local hospital and yet, his patients loved

him. My grandmother was his favorite fan. I knew to find someone that had not been completely brainwashed to the 'good ol' boys' way of medicine. I found him!!! He was a good-hearted man and he helped me bridge over to my Lyme specialist, out of state. I requested a nebulizer and he wrote the nebulizer prescription for me. Then, by God's grace, the lady at the medical supply store couldn't find a code to use in the system bcs they were trying to avoid the word Lyme.

So, instead, she gave me a discount to buy it for cash. That nebulizer, together with the glass container I ordered from Amazon, was like 'PURE GOLD' to me during those dark days. Hence, my journey led me to nebulizing THYME & other essential oils, as well as, 5000 ppm of colloidal silver, nebulized for my mycoplasma. (The 5000 ppm colloidal silver was thanks to side advice from a high-ranking retired military officer/physician) ....

I have nebulized several oils with distilled water over the past 6 years......(CBD, CLOVE, THYME, FRANKINCENSE, 'GERM FIGHTER blend from Plant Therapy, as well as, LEMON, and OREGANO)....I buy all my oils from Plant Therapy, except OREGANO. I buy OREGANO on Amazon from Zane Hellas, located in Greece. I DO NOT RECOMMEND THIS TREATMENT TO ANYONE!!!! I'm only sharing my story. You must know that if nebulized too strong or improperly, it could damage your lungs. ASK YOUR NATUROPATH MD before trying this.

WARNING: I am not a doctor. I am not recommending this. It is not advice and nothing I say is meant to be for prevention, diagnosis, treatment, nor cure. I'm just sharing my journey through Lyme disease and how these oils have helped me for educational purposes .

NOTE: One TV network reported that poison control calls related to EO have doubled in past 8 years, since the essential oil industry has made oils so accessible to the public.. (Is that true or fake news? I'm not sure whether that is true or just media conforming to 'The big boys' pressure to broadcast 'fear', I'm not sure.

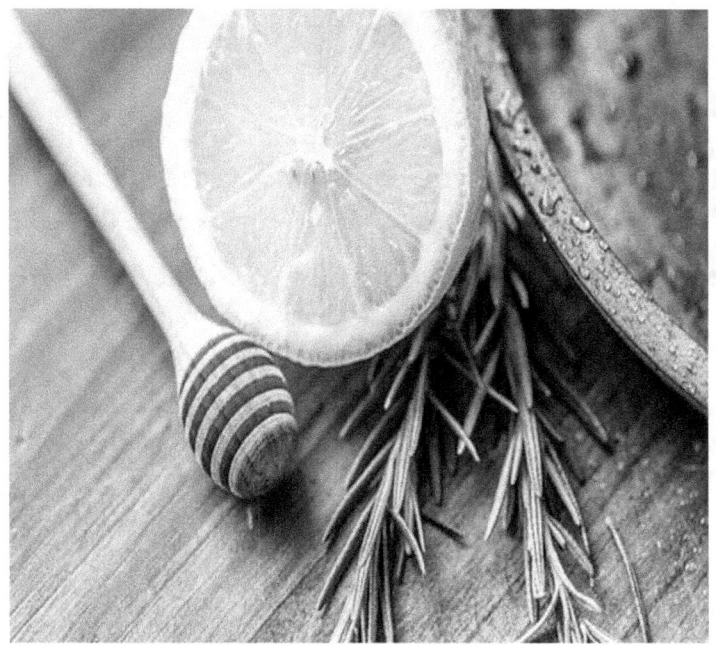

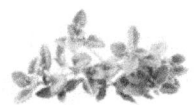

"I am always doing that which I cannot do, in order that I may learn how to do it".
~Pablo Picasso

BONUS SECTION TWO
Thyme Recipes

Here are a few special personally crafted recipes that I love and want to share…I'm proud to use the fresh aromatic Thyme grown in my own garden in these recipes……Thyme is noted for its clean fragrance. In fact, researching history back to the days of Roman soldiers walking the streets, it was actually a compliment when someone said, "Mmmm…You smell of 'thyme'.

Today we use thyme to flavor potatoes, lentils, Mediterranean dishes, lamb, cheeses, soups, European stews, etc... The list can go on and on. Thyme sprigs are often found in the kitchen windows of many European cottages and in the condiment trays of fine bars… I love both the fresh and the dried form of thyme from my garden.

So, with no further ado, I want to share some of my random recipes using THYME. The recipes range from Thyme biscuits to Thyme oils to cleaning solutions using Thyme. I hope you enjoy them. The one I use the most is the LYME BULLET. It is my 'go to' instead of chemical, manmade antibiotics of which I avoid like the plague. I have already shared this recipe, but I'll share it again in this section. It was/is potent for me.

FYI: Historically, political figures and their officers ate thyme just before sitting down to eat a meal. They believed that thyme would offset anyone's attempt to possible poison their food. Thyme is said to neutralize some poisons.

….GOT THYME?

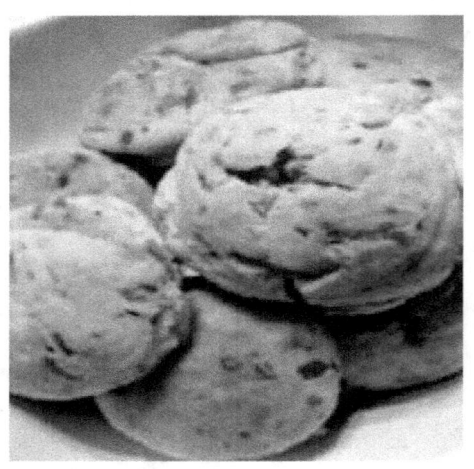

Kentucky Thyme & Cheddar Biscuits

2 cups all-purpose flour
1 tablespoon baking powder
2 teaspoon Himalayan salt
1 Tbsp extra virgin olive oil
1/3 cup shortening
3/4 cup shredded cheddar cheese
3 tablespoons chopped fresh thyme AND 6 drops of Thyme EO
2 tablespoons chopped fresh chives
1 cup milk +/- (Use as needed for proper dough consistency)

Kentucky Thyme & Cheddar Biscuits (Con't)

DIRECTIONS

Preheat oven to 430 degrees F.

Mix with a whisk, flour, baking powder, and salt in a bowl.

Add 1/3 cup of shortening. Use a pastry blender to cut the mixture until it is crumbs.

Add cheddar cheese, thyme and chives into flour crumb mixture

Stir in milk to form a soft dough.

Pour dough out onto a floured cutting board or table surface.

Flour hands well before kneading dough.

Knead dough until smooth consistency for approximately 20 times into a ball

Roll thick dough ball with a wooden rolling pin into a 1" thick sheet of dough.

Use cookie cutter to cut biscuit shapes. Make sure to use dough 'scraps' by re-kneading them and then cutting additional biscuits, in order to maximize dough.

Place cut biscuits onto ungreased cookie sheet.

Bake in preheated oven until golden brown, about 15 minutes.

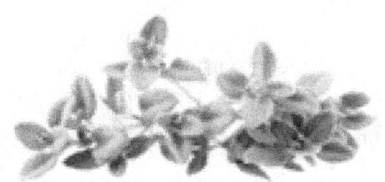

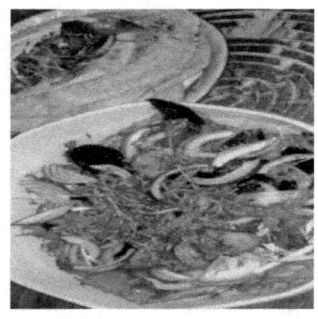

Lebanese Style Thyme Salad

Spring Salad Greens or Arugula
Fresh Thyme
1 large red/white onion (cut in long thin slices)
4 green onions chopped
3-4 mandarin oranges peeled/pulled apart and placed in
salad greens
3 Tbsp. Extra Virgin Olive Oil
1 lemon squeezed over greens
Himalayan Salt to taste
Pita bread

DIRECTIONS: I ozone all vegetables, fruits, & meat
before preparing. The ozone process kills pathogens. (I
purchased a small ozone machine from Amazon.com.
and use it constantly on all vegetables, fruits, and meats
before I prepare them to cook or eat.) Cut & toss
ingredients together. This salad will have somewhat of
a healthy bitter taste with the fresh thyme. It is an
acquired taste for some. In Lebanon, it is normally
eaten with pita bread. I, sometimes, add mandarin
oranges for a sweet element. Traditional Lebanese
thyme salads do not contain mandarins.

Thyme Infused Salad Oil

Break sprigs of fresh thyme, wash well, and stuff into a glass bottle full of Extra Virgin Olive Oil. Let infuse for 2 weeks before using. This will make an excellent thyme oil for salads.

Lemon Thyme Infused Oil

Find yourself a beautiful oil bottle with a cork or top that will keep it sealed well. Clean and sanitize your bottle.

1 lemon zested (peeled with only the zest)
3 sprigs of Thyme from your garden
Large bottle of Extra Virgin Olive Oil

Put the zest peel of 1 lemon into the bottle
Add 3 sprigs of thyme to the bottle
Fill the bottle with Extra Virgin Olive Oil

Cap & Label
Put in dark cool area for 2 weeks. Over the 2 weeks, the oils from the zest of the lemon skin and the thyme sprig will infuse with the olive oil. After 2 weeks, you will have a beautiful blend of infused Lemon/Thyme Oil….

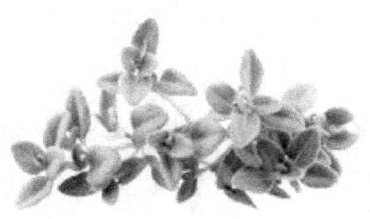

"Believe you can and you're way there."
~T. Roosevelt

The Rub Recipe

½ Tbsp. Paprika
3Tbsp. Pepper
3Tbsp. Cayenne Pepper
3Tbsp Dried Oregano (Greek)
6Tbsp. Garlic powder
6Tbsp.Onion powder
6Tbsp.Dried Thyme
6Tbsp.Himalayan Salt

DIRECTIONS
Mix well and store in sealed container. Add 1 Tbsp. of olive oil to mixture before using on meat.

Thyme Herbal Tea

Dried thyme OR fresh thyme (Thymus vulgaris)
1 ¼ cup of distilled water
Himalayan salt
1 tsp raw honey

DIRECTIONS
Place 1 ¼ cup of distilled water in pan and bring to boil. Turn boiling water to low and simmer. Place Dried Thyme tea bags or bulk Thyme into boiling water. (Fresh thyme will require same directions as dried thyme).

Simmer for 10-15 minutes. Add pinch of salt and 1 tsp of honey.
Pour into cup and ENJOY!!!

Scrambled Eggs With Thyme

2 Eggs
Couple pinches of dried thyme mixed into the eggs

Scramble eggs and mix the dried thyme throughout as you scramble them. Sprinkle top with additional dried thyme.

Thyme Milk…. (It's Fantastic!!)

1 cup warm almond milk (Can also use coconut milk)
Fresh thyme
1 tsp Manuka honey

DIRECTIONS
Heat milk. Add fresh thyme. Let simmer for 15 minutes. Stir in 1 tsp of Manuka honey. ENJOY!!!

Thyme Simple Syrup

1 cup distilled water
1 cup organic sugar
¾ cup thyme sprigs

Put in saucepan and bring to boil. Let cool and then remove the thyme sprigs. Bottle, Label, & Store. Great to use in cocktail recipes.

Holiday Bourbon Thyme

1 1.2 oz Hudson Baby Bourbon (100% corn)
½ oz thyme simple syrup
1 ¾ tbsp cherry preserves
¾ oz lemon juice
2 dashes Angostura Bitters

Serve in a rocks glass
Garnish with thyme sprig & cherries

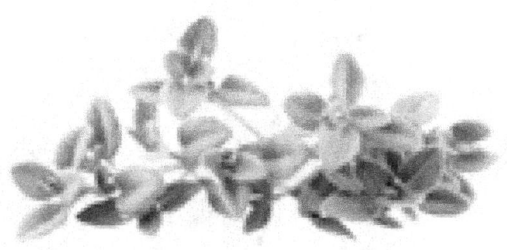

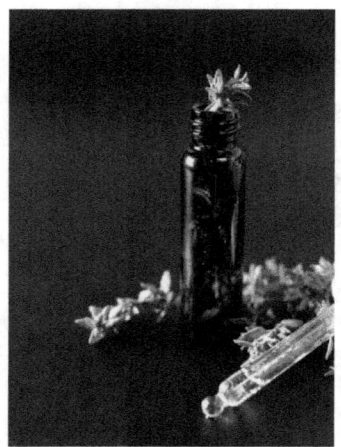

ESSENTIAL OIL WARNING

Do not use thyme essential oil if you have high blood pressure, are pregnant, or have sensitive skin. All topical applications need to be tested in a skin patch test first.

Remember, when blending thyme, keep in mind that it is a middle note and it will blend fantastically with lemon, lavender, pine, bergamot, grapefruit, eucalyptus, and rosemary. Moreover, using a blend that attains the synergistic formula of thymol, carvacrol, and eugenol components is very healing.

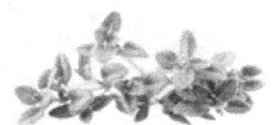

THYME INFUSED HONEY

1 clean food jar with lid
Bunch of thyme -(washed)
Organic raw honey

Fill the jar full of thyme sprigs. Cover the thyme with organic raw honey. Make sure no bubbles are in the honey and the thyme is completely covered with honey. Seal your jar and sit in a sunny window for at least 2-3 weeks. Test the infusion process by tasting the honey at the end of the 2nd week. If it tastes of thyme, then it is ready for the thyme sprigs can be removed from the honey, but don't necessarily have to be if they are under the honey and not exposed to air.
Make sure to label the jar 'INFUSED HONEY WITH THYME'.

This infused honey should last for several months.

Great to use in cough syrup recipes and to make cough drops or cough lollipops or to use in a multitude of recipes.

THYME FOR LEMON LOLLIPOPS

1 cup granulated sugar
1/3 cup water
 Put in saucepan and heat to 320 degrees
Then, blend:
¼ tsp citric acid
2 ½ tsp of fresh lemon zest
1 ½ tsp fresh thyme leaves broken up by hand

Add to heated syrup mixture in saucepan and pour into a heat proof measuring cup.

Pour mixture from measuring cup to pan. Pour 1 – 1 ½" circles on the outsides of the pan only so that you can lay the lollipop sticks inward. They should harden and be ready to enjoy within 45 minutes.

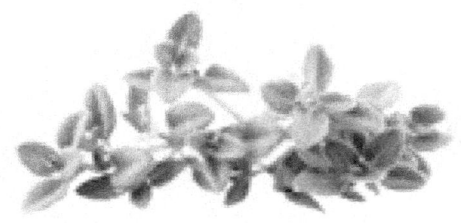

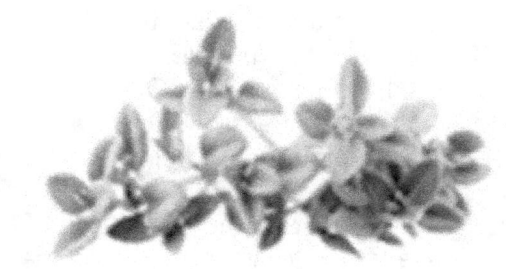

Ear Infection Essential Oil Blend

3 drops of thyme essential oil
2 drops tea tree (melaleuca EO)
1 drop lavender EO
1 drop oregano EO
1 tsp black seed oil

Blend EO together well and then add 1 tsp of black seed oil. Message this total blend around the outside of the ear area, including neck area below, in front of, and behind the outer ear. Rub oil into jawbone area, as well as cheekbone area…. This blend ensures the healing components of essential oils work synergistically. The constituents of thymol, carvacrol, and eugenol are very healing components…. Black seed oil is cumin oil, which is mentioned, medicinally, in the book of Leviticus in the Holy Bible and, mentioned in the Quran. Lay a warm dry compress on area after gently massaging oils around the ear area.

Thyme Tincture for RESPIRATORY

Fresh thyme
TITO's handmade vodka (at least 40% alcohol content)
Clean jar/lid

Cut the thyme into tiny sections and fill your empty bottle/jar.
Cover the herbs with the vodka. Make sure you have a 50/50 mix of herbs & alcohol. Also make sure the herbs are covered completely with vodka. Label the bottle, put a lid on and sit the bottle in a dark cool place for at least 3-4 weeks. Once the tincture is ready for use, then I strain the thyme material out and the remaining liquid can be used 1 tsp 3x daily for a cough and respiratory issues

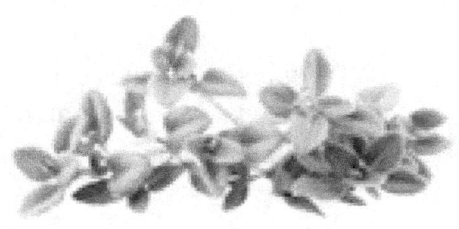

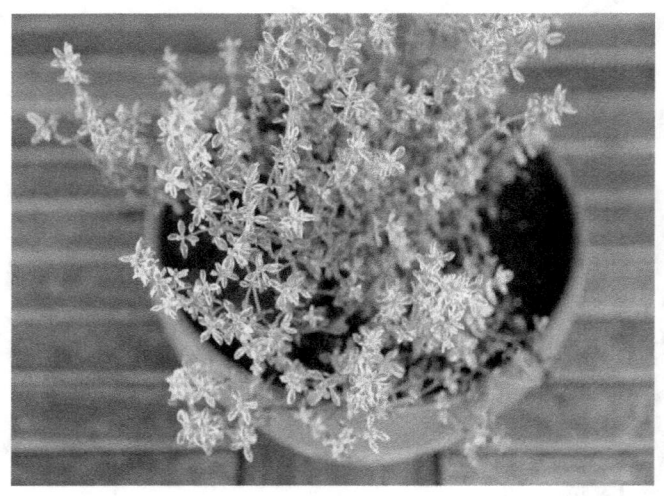

Thyme & Honey Essential Oil Cough Syrup

2 cups distilled water
1 cup Manuka honey
Fresh thyme

Place water in small pan and place on burner. Heat water until it reaches the boiling point. Remove from heat and add the Thyme. Cover and let sit for 10 minutes or until cooled. Whisk in the honey until dissolved. You can store this in a glass jar with lid. cough syrup should last up to 2 months. Cough syrup must be refrigerated. Take 1 tsp as needed to suppress cough.

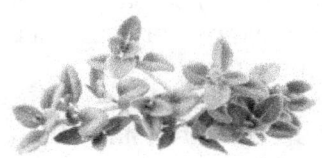

"I spritz Lavender essential oil, diluted in distilled water on my pillowcases & sheets every night"
~K. Badea

Massage Oil for Aching Muscles

6 drops - Thyme
4 drops - Peppermint
4 drops - Lavender
3 drops - Marjoram
10 ml - Black Seed Oil

Blend essential oils first, then add to the black seed oil. Massage aching muscle area. Half of this blend can be added to the bath water. (You can save the other half for your next bath.)   Those with sensitive skin should be very careful and use with precautionary measures.   Peppermint smells great, but it can be a skin irritant for some people. Should you need to dilute the strength of the oils, just add more carrier oil (Black Seed Oil).

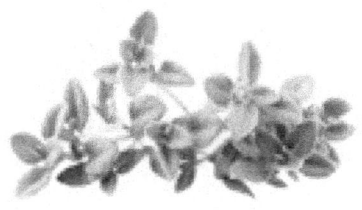

"There is no medicine like hope, no incentive so great, and no tonic so powerful as expectation of something tomorrow."
~Orison Swett Marden

Full Body Massage for Wellness Purposes

I use black seed oil as my massage carrier oil and my husband GENEROUSLY pours drops of THYME, TEA TREE, GERM FIGHTER BLEND, OREGANO, FRANKINCENSE & CLOVE essential oils on my body with the black seed oil. He then rubs them in very well from shoulders to feet, front and back. We have done this nightly for 5 years now. This is part of my successful healing journey that I hope to share with the world... I attribute much of my wellness to 'essential oils'.

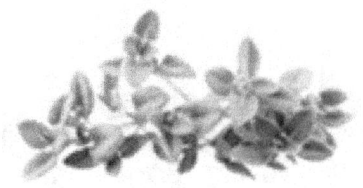

Skin Blemish Mask

2 drops of thyme essential oil
1 drop of lemon essential oil
1 tbsp sour cream
1 tsp unfiltered honey (optional)

Put all ingredients into a blender. Blend well for 2 minutes. Clean face well and put mask mixture on entire face. Leave on for 15 minutes and then rinse face well. Be aware of photosensitivity with the Lemon oil in the mixture, so stay out of the sun afterwards.

Thyme Bath Salts

½ cup Epsom Salt
½ cup Dead Sea Salt
¼ cup Dried Lavender Flowers
20 drops Thyme Essential Oil
5 drops Lemon Essential Oil
5 drops Lavender Essential Oil

DIRECTIONS:
In bowl, add epsom salt, Dead Sea salt and toss/blend.

OPTIONAL: Natural color additive: 1/8 tsp. ultramarine violet mica to tint salts
OPTIONAL: 1/8 tsp of violet color mica for salts.

Toss & blend well to make sure the color of salts is consistent and blended in well.
Add Lavender flowers & toss easily to blend.

In a separate small bottle, blend thyme, lemon,
and lavender essential oils.
Place cap on the bottle and shake well.
Pour bottle of blended oils into the salt &
lavender mixture.
Toss easily and blend well.
Place in nice jar with lid and label.

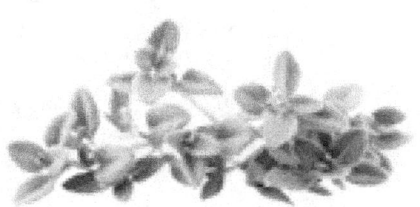

Snoring? Try Thyme

Some use thyme essential oil before bedtime by applying 1-2 drops on the bottom of your feet to prevent snoring. Yes, that's what I said.
(I tend to use essential oils much more ABUNDANTLY than 1-2 drops.)

Thyme Antifungal Cream

1 cup Shea Butter
1 Tbsp. EV Olive Oil
25 drops of Thyme Essential Oil (Thymus zygis…39-74% thymol)
5 drops Tea Tree Oil

DIRECTIONS:
Mix 1 cup of shea butter with 1 Tbsp extra virgin olive oil and whip with blender.
Add 25 drops of thyme essential oil and 5 drops of tea tree oil
Whip until smooth
Pour into a glass jar with lid and label.
This is a great recipe for rubbing on feet or other skin areas that have fungal infections. Use disposable gloves to apply to fungal areas of skin.

Throat Spray for Snoring

Amazon sells a brand of throat spray for snoring. It is comprised of a multitude of essential oils. I have not found any studies to prove its efficacy. However, it is called, 'Helps Stop Snoring'. It is comprised of THYME ESSENTIAL OIL, along with various other essential oils. Check it out. I have not used it.

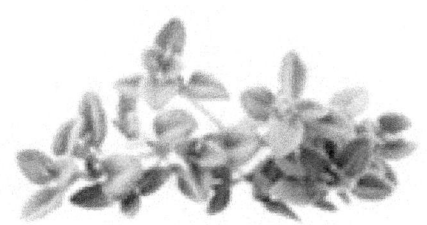

"I only use essential oils for perfumes."
~Jessica Capshaw

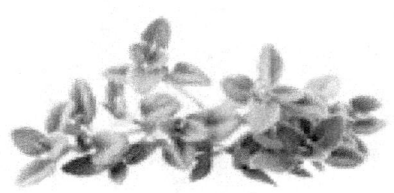

*Knowing others is intelligence; knowing yourself is
true wisdom. Mastering others is strength;
mastering yourself is true power."*
~Lao-Tzu

Thyme Essential Oil Cleaning Solutions

Thyme Antimicrobial Spray for Toothbrush

20 drops thyme essential oil
½ cup distilled water
2 ½ tsp baking soda
1 tsp hydrogen peroxide (3%)

Put in 4oz spray bottle. Tighten lid and shake. Spray on toothbrush to kill microbes lurking inside the bristles. Let this spray mixture stay on the brush until the next use. Before using it, rinse brush thoroughly.

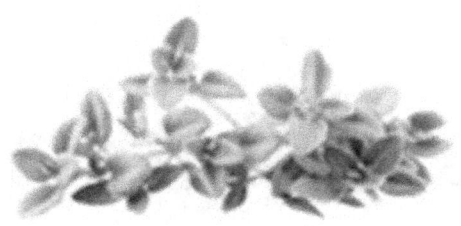

It's THYME to Clean the Oven

3/4 cup salt
1/2 cup borax
1 box baking soda (16 oz)
1/2 cup water
1 cup white vinegar
15 drops thyme essential oil
15 drops lemon or lemongrass essential oil

This mixture will clean a dirty neglected oven... You can always add more salt for scrubbing. Use steel wool to scrub oven with this mixture.

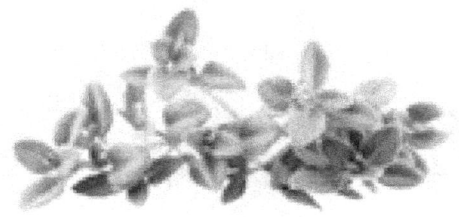

Pet Maintenance

Dog Flea Spray Recipe

(DO NOT USE ON CATS OR OTHER ANIMALS!!!)
20 drops of Thyme Essential Oil
12 drops Catnip EO
12 drops of Citronella EO
6 drops of Lemon Essential Oil
6 drops of Lime Essential Oil
5 drops of Pine Essential Oil
4 drops of Melaleuca EO
3 drops of Austrian Fir EO
3 drops of Siberian Fir EO
2 drops of Cilantro EO
1 4 oz dark spray bottle
Distilled water

DIRECTIONS
Fill 4 oz. spray bottle HALF way with distilled water.
Drop each amount of essential oils from above list into
the 2 oz of distilled water. Then, continue filling bottle to
the top and place spray top on the bottle well. Shake
and it's ready to spritz on your dog.

*"The protection of THYME I seek, for this dog
sweet & meek"*
~Sparky (Just teasing..lol)

Disclaimer

I am not a professional licensed health practitioner and in no way is anything herein meant to prevent, diagnose, treat, nor cure a health condition. This report is for educational purposes only. This data is not considered to be complete and is not guaranteed to be accurate. One must see a licensed health practitioner for all health issues. In addition, all persons, corporations, suppliers, educational venues, etc.... mentioned within this report, are not affiliated with me personally in any way. I am merely mentioning certain entities for educational purposes only. One must decide independently what sources they will use as authorities in their own practice. I, nor any entity herein, takes responsibility for any of the sources, websites, directions, information, protocols, nor any portion, herein, that I have chosen to write about within this book.

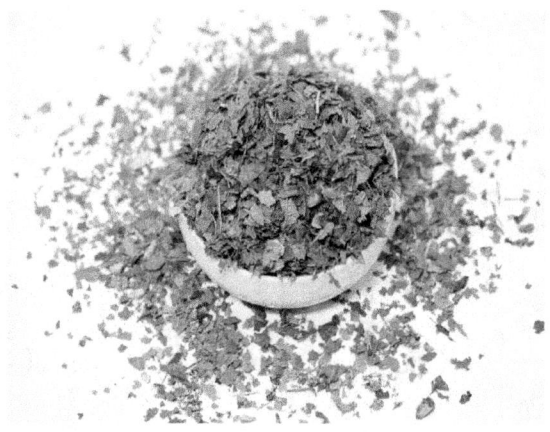

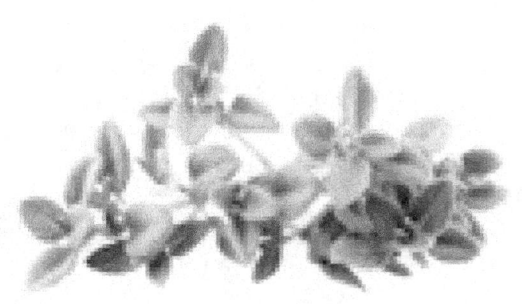

"All the advice in the world will never help you until you help yourself."
~Fred Van Amburgh

My Closing Words

I will end this book with another reminder to always use essential oils from a reputable supplier that is open to showing you GC/MS data on each oil. If you buy wholesale, this is paramount to making sure that your clients get the best therapeutic care possible. No one wants to take the risk of adulterated essential oil products. Deal with only dependable sources when purchasing essential oils. Always be aware of the safety precautions of the oils you use by keeping a good reference library on essential oil safety. In addition, always protect your divine essential oils by keeping them in a dark, cool location with the lids properly tightened, to decrease the oxidation factor

I hope I leave you with the desire to learn even more about each individual essential oil. Never stop learning and always be open to trying new essential oils. Your customers depend upon your expertise and knowledge. I have pledged to continue to always stay updated on the latest information in the essential oil industry…

Perhaps we shall meet one day in an essential oil distillery, in an Aromatherapy conference, or on a mountain high where the herbs are growing in some exotic foreign country… Hopefully, we will find 'thyme' to stop and smell the herbs along life's journey… I have added a bonus section for those interested in learning more about the field of aromatherapy. I have also added a second bonus section for thyme recipes, including culinary, medicinal, and body care recipes. I hope you find the recipes to be very helpful, as well as, fun to make.

Experimenting with essential oils has become addictive for me. I am sold on the healing benefits of essential oils …

I hope that you now see why I said, "Thyme in your garden can be quite different than thyme in mine". It all depends on the Chemotype and the many variables of plant production. It all depends on your aspirations for the beautiful plants that you chose to grow in your garden…. What will you do with them?

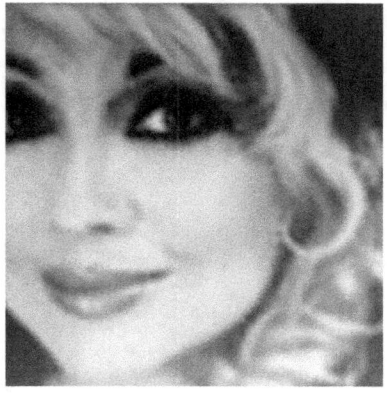

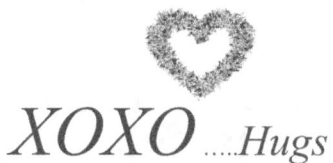

XOXO ….*Hugs*

"Remember, your 'thyme', is very valuable…. Use it wisely."

~Karen Badea

Karen L. Badea

About the Author

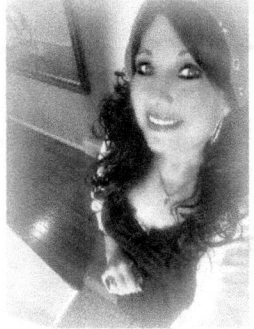

"Blessings to you & your family. May you find quality thyme in your garden......."

Karen Badea is a Certified Aromatherapist with an insatiable interest in alternative medicine. She is especially interested in using essential oils internally for medicinal purposes. Karen has studied biological sciences and graduated Eastern Ky University. She is also a Certified Hypnotherapist and a graduate of Hypnosis Motivational Institute in Tarzana, CA. In addition, Karen is also a Reiki Master. She has self-studied a plethora of alternative healing modalities, with plans of completing a certification as a Master Herbalist. Her motivation to learn alternative medicinal options, stems from her diagnosis in 2013 of Chronic Lyme Disease. She has fought all odds to stay alive and to find a state of remission from Lyme & coinfections. Karen says if not for essential oils, she wouldn't be alive today.

Karen was a US Merchant Marine and worked on the cruise ships for years. She married her husband, Daniel, in Romania 14 years ago and is 'Nana' to five beautiful grandchildren. Karen lives with her husband in Central Kentucky. She had a humble childhood, growing up in rural Kentucky on a family farm that has been in her family since the late 1800's.

Karen's parents raised tobacco, beef cattle, and also bred Belgian horses, in addition, to their full-time careers outside of the farm. She loves gardening and prides herself in foraging medicinal weeds for her backyard wild garden…Karen hopes that her Farmacy Cabinet Series will help you to love the potency of plants as much as she does…

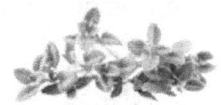

ESSENTIAL OIL DISTILLATION EQUIPMENT
MANUFACTURER THAT I WILL BE PURCHASING
MY EQUIPMENT FROM IN THE NEAR FUTURE.

Here is the information on the company in Portugal that
sells various copper distillery equipment. They even
have a training module on essential oils, Aromatherapy,
Hydrolats, and Perfumes. In my opinion, these are the
most attractive stills that I've found. They are gorgeous!
I'm buying the 5 gallon still. I can't wait to own my first
distillation system.
(http://www.copper-
alembic.com/ns/cms.php?id_cms_category=2)

Iberian Coppers S.A.
Avenida Dr. Francisco Sanches, Nº 22
Tuído
4930-327 VALENÇA
Portugal
Phone: +351 251 823 370
http://www.copper-alembic.com/ns/

DISCLAIMER: I am not endorsing this equipment. I'm
only sharing for educational purposes. You must do
your own research before purchasing your equipment. I
take no responsibility for this companies products and
nor do they take responsibility for my claims. I am just
sharing what I'm doing with essential oils. Its sad that
we have to put so many disclaimers, but there is always
that ONE that requires people to have to do
this…Blessings and I hope you enjoy their website. I
love their website!!

Bibliography

[1] Vegas Vitamins, Vitamin Spot, (2015), Essential Oils All-Natural Healing, All-Natural Healing with Essential Oils, http://vegasvitaminspot.com/essential-oils-all-natural-healing/

[2] Unknown Author, The Old Farmer's Almanac, (2015), Thyme, http://www.almanac.com/plant/thyme

[3] The Taunton Press, Fine Gardening, (2015), Woolly Thyme, Thymus pseudolanuginosus, http://www.finegardening.com/woolly-thyme-thymus-pseudolanuginosus

[4] Stewart, David, Healing Oils of The Bible, (2003), Care Publications, April 25, 2003

[5] Unknown Author, Green Earth Institute, (2015), About Thyme, Thymus vulgaris, http://greenearthinstitute.org/index.php?main_page=document_general_info&cPath=1_62&products_id=1557

[6] Ibid

[7] en.wikipedia.org, Hippocratic Corpus, November 2015

[8] Nordqvist C., Medical News Today, (Pub. Sept. 2013, Last Updated Sept 2014), What Are the Benefits of Thyme? http://www.medicalnewstoday.com/articles/266016.php

[9] Ibid

[10] Crystal, Ellie, Crystal Links, (2015), Ancient Egyptian Medicine, http://www.crystalinks.com/egyptmedicine.html

[11] Ryman, D., Daniele Ryman, (2014), Thyme, http://aromatherapybible.com/thyme/

[12] Holt, Douglas Burner, Essential Oils, http://younglivingessentialoils.com.au/thyme-essential-oil-aromatherapy/, May 21, 2013

[13] Cantwell, Marite, Reid, Michael, Department of Plant Sciences, University of California, Davis Division of Agriculture and Natural Resources, http://postharvest.ucdavis.edu/pfvegetable/Herbs/
[14] Stahl-Biskup and Saez, (2014) Thyme: The Genus Thymus Summary, London and New York, Taylor & Francis
[15] Pappas R., Essential Oil University (2015), About Essential Oil University, http://essentialoil.university/about/
[16] Schnaubelt, Kurt, Dr., Roots: Thyme Chemotypes From Provence, http://www.kurtschnaubelt.com/, November 19, 2012
[17] Tisserand and Young, (2014) Essential Oil Safety, 2nd Edition, Edinburgh et al., Churchill Livingstone Elsevier, www.elsevierhealth.com, p.448, 450
[18] Martin N., LSHC, CRTS, Experience Essential Oils.com, (2015), Thyme Oil Supports Healthy Immune and Digestive Systems, http://www.experience-essential-oils.com/thyme-oil.html
[19] Tisserand and Young, (2014) Essential Oil Safety, 2nd Edition, Edinburgh et al., Churchill Livingstone Elsevier, www.elsevierhealth.com, p.448, 450
[20] Ibid.
[21] Ibid.
[22] Robineau, L., Farmacopea vegetal caribeña, en da-caribe, 2007 - Materia médica, Vegetable. 485 pages
[23] Ibid
[24] Ibid
[25] Axtell, B.L., FAO AGRICULTURAL SERVICES BULLETIN No. 94 FOOD AND AGRICULTURE ORGANIZATION OF THE UNITED NATIONS, Rome, 1992 Intermediate Technology Development Group, Rugby, UK, M-17, ISBN 92-5-103128-2, (c)

FAO
https://www.erowid.org/archive/rhodium/chemistry/3bas
e/safrole.plants/moc/distillation.html, 1992
[26] Ibid (Stahl)
[27] Adams, Case, Naturopath, Heal Naturally,
http://www.realnatural.org/
[28] Kline, L., Kline Krest Certified Organic Produce
Farm in Michigan, (2015), ORAC Values Chart,
http://www.klinekrestcertifiedorganicproduce.com/Kline
KrestOracValuesChart.htm
[29] Salmalian Hajar et al, Comparative effect of thymus
vulgaris and ibuprofen on primary dysmenorrhea: A
triple-blind clinical study, http://www.ncbi.nlm.nih.gov/
[30] Ibid (Stahl)
[31] Ibid (Stahl)
[32] Soković, et al., PubMed, 2009, Chemical
composition of essential oils of Thymus and Mentha
species and their antifungal activities., Jan 7;14(1):238-
49. doi: 10.3390/molecules14010238
[33] Kavanaugh et al., PubMed, Selected Antimicrobial
Essential Oils Eradicate Pseudomonas spp. And
Staphylococcus aureus Biofilms,
http://www.ncbi.nlm.nih.gov/pmc/articles/PMC3346404
/[34] Hull, J, Dr. Jennifer Starr Hull, Alternative &
Nutrition, 2011, How to Get the Bugs Out,
http://www.janethull.com/newsletter/0107/how_to_get_t
he_bugs_out_1.php
[35] Mercola, Joseph, Dr., Mercola.com, 'Herbal Oil:
Thyme Oil Benefits and Uses', December 06, 2015
[36] Sajed et al., Journal of Ethnopharmacology,
Volume 145, Issue 3, 13 February 2013, Zataria
multiflora Boiss. (Shirazi thyme)—An ancient
condiment with modern pharmaceutical uses, Pages

686–698,
http://www.sciencedirect.com/science/article/pii/S03788
7411200852
[37] Alizadeh et al., PubMed, Commun Agric Appl Biol
Sci. 2010;75(4):761-7. Antifungal activity of some
essential oils against toxigenic Aspergillus species,
http://www.ncbi.nlm.nih.gov/pubmed/21534488
[38] Mohammed Nasir1, Ketema Tafess1, Dawit Abate2
'Antimicrobial potential of the Ethiopian Thymus
schimperi essential oil in comparison with others against
certain fungal and bacterial species', 'Total Synthesis of
(±)-Vaticanol A', Synfacts, 2014
[39] Grieve M., Botanical.com, 2014, Thyme Garden,
https://www.botanical.com/botanical/mgmh/t/thygar16.h
tml
[40] Summerly J., PreventDisease.com, 2015, 20 Health
Benefits of Thyme Oil, Health Impact
News,http://healthimpactnews.com/2015/20-health-
benefits-of-thyme-oil/
[41] Lyth, Geoff,
http://www.quinessence.com/blog/thyme-sweet-
essential-oil
[42] Zu Y1, Yu H, Liang L, Fu Y, Efferth T, Liu X, Wu
N, National Center for Biotechnology Information,
Article Title: Result Filters, Publisher: U.S. National
Library of Medicine, Date Accessed: December06,2015,
http://www.ncbi.nlm.nih.gov/pubmed/20657472
[43] Holt, Douglas, Young Living Essential Oils
Australia,
[44] Horowitz, Len, Dr., DeVita, Sebina, Dr.,
ANTHRAX NATURAL CURES, December 06, 2015,
http://www.theforbiddenknowledge.com/hardtruth/anthr
ax_cures.htm

[45] Holt, Douglas, Young Living Essential Oils Australia, 'What Everyone Ought to Know About Thyme Essential Oil - Young […]', Electronically Published: May 21, 2013, Date Accessed: December 06, 2015

[46] Seward M., Healthy Focus, (2015), The 9 Most Powerful Antifungal Essential Oils, http://healthyfocus.org/the-9-most-powerful-antifungal-essential-oils/

[47] [Seung-Joo Lee a, Katumi Umano b, Takayuki Shibamoto c, Kwang-Geun Lee d,* Department of Food Science and Technology, Dongguk University, 3-26 Pil-dong, Chung-gu, Seoul 100-715, Republic of Korea b Takata Koryo Co. Ltd., 22-2 7-Chome, Tsukaguchi-Honmachi, Amagasaki, Hyogo-Pref. 661, Japan c Department of Environmental Toxicology, University of California, Davis, CA 95616, USA a Korea Food Research Institute, Seongnam-si, Republic of Korea. Received 4 May 2004; received in revised form 27 May 2004; accepted 27 May 2004]

[48] Lee S et al, ScienceDirect.com, 2004, Identification of volatile components in basil (Ocimum basilicum L.) and thyme leaves (Thymus vulgaris L.) and their antioxidant properties, http://eurekamag.com/pdf/031/031793310.pdf

[49] Inouye et al., OxfordJournals.org., 2001, Antibacterial activity of essential oils and their major constituents against respiratory tract pathogens by gaseous contact, http://jac.oxfordjournals.org/content/47/5/565.full

[50] Ibid

[51] Unknown Author, HerbWisdom.com, 2014, Thyme Thymus, http://www.herbwisdom.com/herb-thyme.html

[52] Ibid

[53] Smith, J., Chakra Balancing Music and Sound Healing for Your Well Being, 4th Chakra, http://balance.chakrahealingsounds.com/4th-chakra/, 2015

[54] Unknown Dylan, Potential new protocol, Cpnhelp.org, December 06, 2015, http://www.cpnhelp.org/potential_new_protocol?page=1 Rose, Jeanne, 'The Aromatherapy Book: Applications and Inhalations', 1992, North Atlantic Books, Berkeley, CA, p. 143

[55] Butje A., distillerdirectory.com, 2015, International Directory of Essential Oil Distillers, https://distillerdirectory.com/

[56] Ibid (Essential Oil Safety/Tisserand)

[57] Ibid

[58] Tisserand, Robert, Robert Tisserand website, December 6, 2015, http://roberttisserand.com/

[59] Mercola, Joseph Dr., http://articles.mercola.com/herbal-oils/thyme-oil.aspx#_edn13, Accessed December 6, 2015, [60] Burfield, Tony, The Adulteration of Essential Oils - and the Consequences to Aromatherapy & Natural Perfumery Practice. Copyright Oct 2003, http://www.users.globalnet.co.uk/~nodice/new/magazine /october/october.htm, December 6, 2015.

[61] Ibid

[62] Butje A., components.aromahead.com, 2015, Component Database from The Aromahead Institute, https://components.aromahead.com/

[63] Directorate Plant Production in collaboration with members of SAEOPA and KARWIL Consultancy, genesisseeds.com, 2009, Thyme Production, Dept Agriculture Forestry & Fisheries, South Africa,

http://www.genesisseeds.com/organicseed/herbs/pdf/Ess
OilsThyme.pdf[64]

Whitaker, A., veriditasbotanicals.com, 2005-2015, Why
Choose Organic? If It's Not Organic It Doesn't Have
the Same Potency, http://veriditasbotanicals.com/about-
us/purity-integrity/

Thank you for your support.

If you enjoyed learning about THYME ESSENTIAL OIL & the herb itself, then check out my next book in this series on OREGANO ESSENTIAL OIL….

I suggest you focus on ONE ESSENTIAL OIL at a time, stock your medicine cabinet with that oil, learn its properties, plant it in a container inside your home or in your garden.

Be able to identify the various varieties of THYME, get comfortable using it in your food and also for medicinal purposes…Repeat this for each essential oil that you add to your WELLNESS CABINET…. Teach your children the healing powers of ORGANIC, NON GMO HERBS…

Amazon will be carrying my entire 'FARMACY CABINET SERIES' and 'Oregano Essential Oil' will be my 2nd book in this series. I hope you dedicate the time to learn.

Thank you from my heart…♡.
May God bless you and your family.

Best wishes,

Karen Badea

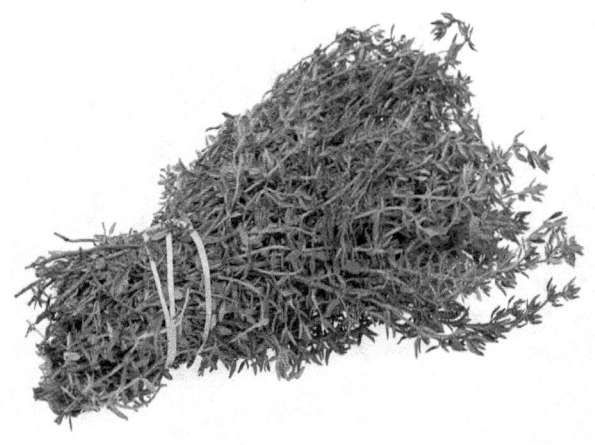

"I came near to the 'doors of death' due to Lyme and its many deadly coinfections. I was forced to fight every second of every day for YEARS, in order to live... I will be forever grateful to those that spread the TRUTH IN MEDICINE and to those that shared NATURE'S HEALING POWERS with me... Share your knowledge on essential oils with everyone you meet because you never know what life you could save."

~Karen Badea

NOTES

NOTES

NOTES

NOTES

www.ingramcontent.com/pod-product-compliance
Lightning Source LLC
Chambersburg PA
CBHW071348280526
45787CB00001B/251